MICROCURRENT STIMULATION

MIRACLE

EYE CURE

D1617590

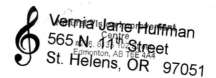

Vernia Jane Huffman
565 N. 11th Street
St. Helens, OR   97051

MICROCURRENT STIMULATION
MIRACLE EYE CURE

Edward C. Kondrot , M.D.

To Dr Curnutt from
Verna Jae Suffun (RN) BSN
MPH

Published by
Nutritional Research Press

Distributed by
North Atlantic Books

The information in this book is meant to complement medical care. Any unusual, sudden, or severe symptoms should be evaluated by an ophthalmologist. The recommendations made from this book, while generally safe and non-toxic, may affect people differently. Therefore it is recommended that individuals with serious eye disease be under the care of a physician.

Published by:
Nutritional Research Press
Carson City, Nevada

Distributed by:
North Atlantic Books
P.O. Box 12327
Berkeley, California 94712

Cover Design by: Behar Fengal Design
Printed in the United States of America

Microcurrent Stimulation; Miracle Eye Cure is distributed by the Society for the Study of native Arts and Sciences, a non-profit educational corporation whose goals are to develop an educational and crosscultural perspective linking various scientific, social and artistic fields; to nurture a holistic view of arts, sciences, humanities, and healing; and to publish and distribute literature on the relationship of mind, body and nature.

ISBN 1-55643-401-4
Library of Congress 99-06970

This book is dedicated to Grace Halloran
for her pioneering spirit in the use of
Microcurrent Stimulation.

Acknowledgments

It is very important to me to let people know of this exciting treatment for macular degeneration called Microcurrent Stimulation (MCS). It can be a miracle cure for thousands of people who suffer from the disability of macular degeneration. It can change the life and sight of many people.

I especially want to thank Grace Halloran for discovering the use of MCS to treat eye disorders. To Sam Snead, who had the courage to undergo MCS for macular degeneration. It was the news report on his treatment that led me to begin MCS.

I thank Dr. Joel Rossen and Dr. Damon Miller for teaching me so much about the role of MCS in the treatment of macular degeneration. I am also very grateful to Dr. Damon Miller for writing the forward and sharing his knowledge and experience using acupuncture to enhance the effects of MCS.

I would also like to thank Cathie Younghans for her hard work in organizing and laying out the manuscript and keeping this project on schedule, my secretaries Marilyn Myrah and Deborah Wessolek for their work in keeping me organized and to my editor Gloria St. John. I thank Christine Faust and Kathleen Brainard-Lee who lovingly administer the MCS treatments in my office.

I am grateful to everyone who worked on the manuscript and contributed their experiences: Joel Rossen, Grace Halloran, Damon Miller, Jeanette Manning, Shiva Pourazima and Robert Eichman.

Last I would like to thank all my patients for letting me be a partner in helping them improve their eyesight.

Edward C. Kondrot, MD

Contents

Foreword by Damon Miller II, M.D., N.D......... . xi

Preface: Another Thief xvii

Introduction 1

Chapter 1
What is Macular Degeneration? 9

Chapter 2
Why doesn't my Doctor know about MCS? 35

Chapter 3
There is Hope. The Grace Halloran Story 45

Chapter 4
Patients tell their Story 57

Chapter 5
The History of Microcurrent Stimulation........... 69

Chapter 6
Can Microcurrent Stimulation Help You? 79

Chapter 7
Getting Acquainted with your Unit 89

Chapter 8
Other uses of Microcurrent Stimulation 121

Chapter 9
Additional Points to Enhance Treatment 149

Chapter 10

Better Nutrition improves your Results 157

Chapter 11

Use Homeopathy and Chelation Therapy 177

Appendix 197
Resources 255

Foreword by
Damon P. Miller II, M.D., N.D.

In this book, Dr. Kondrot presents a thorough and thoughtful evaluation of the use of Microcurrent Stimulation therapy in the treatment of various retinal diseases. He is the first to point out that Microcurrent Stimulation (MCS) is not a "magic bullet" and it is not a cure for Age Related Macular Degeneration or other similar conditions that affect the eye. Still, it is the only therapy that has been found that has produced significant and lasting improvements in the vision of the vast majority of those who have used it, and as such, it truly is a miracle therapy. In this and in his previous book, *Healing the Eye the Natural Way, Alternative Medicine and Macular Degeneration*, Dr. Kondrot has also been very thorough and insistent in his discussion of the importance of a healthy lifestyle, and he goes to great length to explain what a healthy lifestyle and healthy nutrition look like for someone with eye disease. He also includes a thoughtful discussion of other therapies such as homeopathy, chelation therapy and acupuncture, which for some people may be useful for the overall treatment of their health and therefore contribute to the treatment of their eye disease. MCS is miraculous, but it is in the context of the treatment of all aspects of a persons health and well-being that it is most effective.

It is an all to common story. A person comes into my office who has been told that they have Macular Degeneration by their Ophthalmologist. The person goes on to tell me that they feel that once the diagnosis was made, it was as though their doctor had written them off, giving them up as hopeless. The person is depressed and fearful, having been told to go home and prepare to be blind. But I know that diseases such as Macular Degeneration, Stargardt Disease, Retinitis Pigmentosa and other degenerative retinal disease are not hopeless. They are very complex and difficult diseases to treat, but they are not hopeless. The treatment is not as simple as a quick surgery or a pill that can be taken once-a-day so that the person can just forget about their disease and go on with their life. The treatment involves and evaluation and adjustment of lifestyle habits that affect health, evaluating nutrition and the use of vitamins and supplements, sometimes in rather large doses, and it involves the use of a technology (MCS) that requires some of their time and attention on a daily basis. Conventional medical wisdom has told these people that they have a progressive and untreatable disease that will eventually leave them without any functional vision. When I see these people devote themselves to the treatment that is laid out for them and recover enough vision that they can get their driver's license again, or when I see a painter recover color vision to the point where they can paint again, or when I see a young and gifted music student recover enough vision that they can read sheet music again, I realize that these treatments truly are miraculous. Even those people who do not show improvement show significant slowing or stoppage in the deterioration of their disease, and if this is all these treatments did, they would be worthwhile.

Microcurrent Stimulation therapy has been used for the treatment of eye disease since the mid 1980's, yet it is still in its infancy. This is not a new technology for conventional medicine, for it has been used in Orthopedic Medicine for the treatment of non-healing bone fractures, in Physical Medicine for the treatment of non-healing soft tissue wounds, and is used extensively in Sports Medicine for its ability to decrease inflammation and swelling in acute musculoskeletal injuries and to speed the healing process in injured tissues. Much deserved credit is given to Grace Halloran who pioneered the use of this technology in the treatment of retinal disease. Grace experienced remarkable improvements in her own vision which had been profoundly impaired at an early age by the disease Retinitis Pigmentosa through the use of Microcurrent Stimulation. She has, since the mid 1980's, made it her life-work to educate others about the use of this technology in the context of a program of total health for the treatment of their eye disease.

The fact that much of the early work using MCS for the treatment of retinal disease was not done by Ophthalmologists has resulted in almost total ignorance by the community of physicians about this remarkable therapy. I offer here a quote from the novel *The Cunning Man* by Robertson Davies , a novel about an unconventional but effective physician :

> *"...there is nothing a professional group mistrusts so nervously as it does anything that appears unconventional, and that has not been thoroughly written up in the journals. It may be quackery. Worse still, it may be effective. and if it is both quackery and effective it is utterly hateful."*

Dr. Kondrot discusses the FDA studies that are taking place that will eventually result in the publication of articles in the journals read by Ophthalmologists, but it is not necessary to wait for this research to be finished. The improvements in the technology that is used to deliver Microcurrent Stimulation have resulted in a new class of devices that are relatively inexpensive and are available with a doctor's prescription for use now. The history of the clinical use of these devices since the 1980's has shown them to be not only effective, but remarkably safe. Microcurrent Stimulation is a miracle whose time has come.

The scientific understanding of how Microcurrent Stimulation works is also in its infancy. When I was in medical school I was taught that the only significant electrical activity that existed in the human body was within the nervous system, with the nerves functioning like wires surrounded by special insulation to carry electrical information to different parts of the body. More recently there has been increasing understanding that there is important electrical activity that occurs at the cellular level, and that there is very significant electrical activity that exists around areas of disease such as tumors, inflammation, or areas with poor blood flow. Björn Nordenström, M.D., a Swedish radiologist and medical researcher at the Karolinska Institute in Sweden, first published his pioneering work in 1983 on the understanding of how these subtle electrical currents functioned in human tissues, and how they might be manipulated to affect healing.[1] In appendices at the end of this book, Dr. Kondrot includes some of the scientific work that is ongoing in an attempt to understand the mechanism of action of Microcurrent Stimulation therapy.

Dr. Kondrot also gives considerable attention to the technology that is needed for these treatments to work at all. Microcurrent Stimulation is not as simple as attaching a couple of wires to a battery and applying some current around your eyes. It is only thanks to the recent advances in the technology associated with this therapy that the treatment is as effective as it is. This book gives careful consideration to the devices used by the practitioners who have been doing this therapy successfully, and should help eliminate some of the confusion that exists about the many electrical stimulation devices on the market that were designed simply as counter-irritant stimulators for pain control, but which have proven ineffective in the treatment of retinal diseases.

This is a book for the millions of people with Macular Degeneration and other degenerative retinal diseases. These diseases are not hopeless, and there is therapy called Microcurrent Stimulation that is remarkabley safe and effective that is available now. It is my prayer that you find out about this therapy, and if you are reading this then my prayer has been answered.

Preface

Another Thief

There is an old adage in ophthalmology about glaucoma. It is known as "The Thief". As America's baby boomers age, a new thief has been appearing with greater and greater frequency, Age Related Macular Degeneration. (ARMD). ARMD is projected to affect nearly 30 million people in the US by the year 2010. If there were such thing as a grand jury of ophthalmology, I would suggest that ARMD be thoroughly investigated and indicted as the new "Thief of Vision".

Age Related Macular Degeneration steals the joy and quality of life for the segment of our society who most deserves to be able to finally take the time to enjoy their lives, the senior citizens. They have put in their years of work and given untold value to us, as educators, inventors, teachers, leaders and parents. Now it is time for us to be able to give back to them so that they can have a life of quality and happiness. ARMD steals their sight, just at a time when they are looking forward to watching their grandchildren grow up. It makes independent living difficult and often impossible.

I am writing this book with a very specific objective. That objective is to save and restore both vision and high quality of life for the many seniors who have been told to plan spending the rest of their lives with constant degeneration of their vision. During my training as an ophthalmologist, I was taught that there was not only no cure for ARMD, there was not even any hope. That is what almost all patients with this disease are told. They are told, go home and plan to lose almost all of your central vision. You will still see movement in the periphery, but eventually, that might be all you see. Eventually, your loss of visual perception is likely to be so severe that you will not be able to drive, see faces, watch TV, sew, or even read. And there is nothing that can be done about it.

For over one year, I have been treating ARMD patients with a new technology, MicroCurrent Stimulation. The vast majority of all the patients I have treated with MicroCurrent have shown measurable improvement and most of the rest have stopped degenerating. This technology works, and that is the message I am compelled to bring to you with this book.

———— Introduction

This is the second in a series of books describing how to treat various eye conditions with natural methods. These include Age-Related Macular Degeneration (ARMD), glaucoma, cataract, and eyestrain. The subject of this book is how Microcurrent Stimulation can successfully reverse Macular Degeneration. Most people who have this disease are so fearful when they hear the diagnosis that they do not even understand what the condition means. Nor do they know how they have got it. And, most distressing of all, they have virtually no information about how to help themselves.

My first book, *Healing the Eye the Natural Way: Alternative Medicine and Macular Degeneration* helped address many of these questions and gave patients a clear 12-step method to improve their vision. This book zooms in on one of the most successful treatments for diseases of the macula and retina, whether they are hereditary or degenerative. This treatment is Microcurrent Stimulation.

In my opinion, Microcurrent Stimulation is a miracle

eye cure. Yet it is very simple. It uses electricity to heal —
a technique that dates back to the ancient Egyptians. In
this book I will take you on a fascinating journey explor-
ing the use of electrical energy in the treatment of disease. We will look at the evolution of this from a device
that was originally designed for another purpose. (If you
have one or even more of the following diseases, there is
hope.) This book will instill hope where doctors have
told you nothing can be done.

> Macular degeneration – wet or dry type
> Diabetic retinopathy
> Vascular retinal disease
> Retinitis pigmentosa
> Juvenile macular degeneration
> Inflammatory retinal disease
> Drug toxicity of the retina

I know that a diagnosis of macular degeneration
strikes fear in the minds of most people. I know this because as an ophthalmologist I give this diagnosis every
day to people who are losing their vision. There is a good
reason for people to feel terror and hopelessness when
they hear this diagnosis from an ophthalmologist who is
unaware of highly effective treatments for this condition.
These treatments include vitamins and minerals, herbs,
homeopathy, and, of course, Microcurrent Stimulation.
Most doctors do not know about these treatments. As a
result, most cases of macular degeneration lead to pro-

gressive deterioration of vision. In fact, Age Related Macular Degeneration is the leading cause of blindness in people over the age of 60. It is estimated that over 13 million people suffer from this condition today and that this number will more than double in the next 10 years. Yet, I maintain that this is an epidemic that can be stopped, and stopping it has become my personal mission and most cherished goal.

My personal and professional journey has been all about healing and helping people. Twenty-five years ago, when I entered medical school, this was my goal as it is today. Specializing in diseases of the eye seemed to be a very promising way to fulfill that goal. I hoped to see diseases that produce blindness and near blindness eliminated in my lifetime. I really believed that it could happen.

As I developed in my practice, I saw that most of my patients did not get better, and many of my treatments, especially those directed at macular degeneration, just delayed the inevitable worsening of their disease. I knew I had to find a better way.

Most of the current therapies used to treat macular degeneration are not effective and in some cases they cause further loss of vision. The new laser therapies that use marking dye are touted as a potential cure. Yet, only a small percentage of patients qualify for this treatment. These are among the 20 percent of patients who have the wet form of macular degeneration. Eighty percent have the dry form, for which there is no treatment. Of those 20 percent with the wet form, only a very few will meet the criteria for laser treatment. Even then, most patients need repeated treatments several times a year, and there is a risk of permanent lose of more vision, since the therapy destroys the healthy tissue along with the diseased retina.

I cannot endorse a treatment that destroys healthy retinal tissue. This treatment violates the first part of the Hippocratic Oath that all physicians must take, the part that instructs us to first and foremost, "do no harm." I am not impressed by treatments that have the potential to harm patients. My ideal treatment is a therapy that reverses pathology using the natural healing ability of the body. We laugh at physicians who, hundreds of years ago who practiced bloodletting and used poisons to treat disease. Future physicians will probably categorize the laser as a folly just as dangerous as bloodletting.

My passion for finding effective, harmless therapies led me to Microcurrent Stimulation (MCS). I became interested in it after reading an article describing its miraculous effect using a device called MicroStim®, invented by Dr. Joel Rossen on the famous golfer Sam Snead. He was suffering from the limitations of macular degeneration, had to quit the senior tour and was no longer able to play golf. After receiving several MCS treatments his vision improved dramatically, and rejoined the tour within one week and was able to play the game he loved. I asked myself whether it was possible that the weak electrical current of Microcurrent Stimulation could reverse the damage of this disease?

4

I was deeply involved in researching the effects of chelation therapy and homeopathy on Macular Degeneration. The results with these modalities were favorable, but most cases required months of treatment before we observed the positive results. I was looking for a method to accelerate the healing process of the body. I also felt that my patients deserved my serious investigation of this procedure. The following day I called Dr. Joel Rossen, president of MicroStim® Technology Incorporated, the manufacturer of the MicroStim® devices, which are used for the treatment of macular degeneration. I asked him for information about this promising procedure. Joel described, in detail, the principles of MCS and the research to date. He said he could not make any claims for his technology when used for macular degeneration. He suggested I evaluate it myself and come to my own conclusions. He said that if I was still interested when I began to see results in my own patients, I might become involved with the proposed future FDA investigations. I had many conversations with Joel and this has lead to a close friendship between us.

The initial clinical trial in my office began with the treatment of ten patients. They were all longstanding patients in my practice with a history of macular degeneration. Most of them had tried other treatments without any improvement of their vision. They were all enthusiastic to try another modality that had the potential to improve their precious gift of sight. This initial trial lasted for several weeks. The results were a pleasant surprise to me. 68% of the patients showed improved vision. The improvement was significant with a range of one to three lines on the vision chart. It was surprising to me that most patients obtained a marked improvement after just a few MCS treatments. Rapid improvement was what I was looking for in a treatment for this condition.

This success convinced me that the results were not a placebo response. Investigators always discuss the placebo response in evaluating any new therapy. It is estimated that 25 to 30% of patients will have favorable results regardless of the effectiveness of the treatment. The patients in my study achieved a much higher rate of improvement than could not possibly be explained by placebo effect. Furthermore, most of them had been involved in previous studies, and none of them had demonstrated a placebo response. My criteria for safe and effective treatment of macular degeneration are as follows: First it adheres to that very important mandate in the Hippocratic Oath — to do no harm. Second it stimulates the natural healing ability of the body without poisoning or destroying tissue. Finally it enables other complementary therapies like homeopathy, vitamin and chelation therapy to heal the body and restore vision. Microcurrent stimulation meets all of my criteria to safely treat macular degeneration.

We are now able to reverse macular degeneration and restore sight! If you or a loved one have this disease and are losing vision, do not give up! Read this book and make the decision to begin this exciting therapy to improve your vision. Explore Microcurrent Stimulation and restore your sight!

Edward C. Kondrot, MD
Pittsburgh, Pennsylvania

This book deals with Microcurrent Stimulation as an alternative treatment for Macular Degeneration. It also discusses lifestyle change and methods that are now being studied within conventional medicine. These have not yet been proven to be effective through scientific research. While trying these approaches, you should remain under the care of your ophthalmologist and have your vision checked periodically. He or she may recommend other treatments, some that may not be available at the time of this writing. If this is the case, you need to evaluate these options. Fortunately, most of the recommendations in this book complement conventional treatment. Your sight is precious, and you need to be assured that you are doing nothing to harm it, as well as everything possible to maintain it.

1 What is Macular Degeneration?

The purpose of this book is to convince you that the use of a therapy called Microcurrent Stimulation will reverse changes to the retina and macula of the eye caused by disorders that cause progressive loss of vision and near blindness. Very few doctors, even if they are ophthalmologists, have heard of this therapy. And, many, sad to say, will tell you that it is not effective. I am saddened by the handicaps that many people live with because they were not informed about natural treatments for their conditions. Microcurrent Stimulation is a miracle cure. The miracle is that it helps restore sight where all hope is lost. It will not necessarily reverse everyone's loss of vision and produce perfect vision. But it will help almost everyone who use it faithfully and who combine it with good nutrition. Before I describe the technique of Microcurrent Stimulation, I want to orient you to the anatomy of the eye as well as review the many conditions that can be helped by Microcurrent Stimulation.

What is Macular Degeneration?

Anatomy of the Eye

To understand the changes that occur in the degeneration of the macula, or macular degeneration, we must understand a little about the anatomy of the eye and the retina. First let us look at the structure in the eye that becomes damaged in macular degeneration, the retina. The retina is responsible for changing light energy into a picture, and sending that image to the brain. It is like the film in a camera. Light enters the camera, is focused on the film and a picture is taken. If you have good quality film you are going to have a great picture, but if the film is damaged then the picture will be of poor quality.

Anatomy of the Retina

There are several important layers of cells that contribute to the functioning of the retina. Each layer is important and must have integrity in order for the eye to see. I want you to become familiar with the names of these important layers and with their function as well as how they are involved in the development of macular degeneration.

The Retinal Layers are:
1)   Sclera
2)   Choroid
3)   Bruch's Membrane
4)   Retinal Pigment cells
5)   Sensory Retina
6)   The Macula

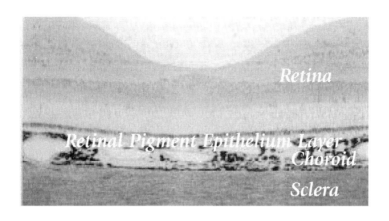

The shell of the eye is called the *sclera*. This consists of a firm hard coat much like the cover of a basketball. It gives the eye a firm shape and helps keep the eye from collapsing. It is often called the "white of the eye." Inside the *sclera* is a vascular structure called the *Choroid*. The *Choroid* supplies the blood and nutrients to the retina. This blood supply is important since the retina has a very high rate of metabolism and needs to be constantly supplied with oxygen, nutrients, and minerals for proper functioning.

Bruch's membrane separates the *Choroid* from the retinal pigment cells. This important membrane protects the retina from the high blood flow of the *Choroid*. We will see later that breaks in this membrane cause blood to leak into the retina causing the wet type of macular degeneration.

The sensory retina is a tissue structure composed of rods and cones and neurons.

What is Macular Degeneration?

It is a layer of cells that provide the foundation or building block of the retina, and is one of the most important layers of cells involved with health of the retina. These cells protect the retina from toxins that can be found circulating in the choroid. The sensory retina is like the film of the camera. It consists of specialized cells and tissue for absorbing light energy and converting it into the electrical impulses that are transmitted to the brain. The rods and cones in the sensory retinal are the specialized elements in which this process is conducted.

The retinal pigment epithelium is a layer of cells that acts as cement, which holds the retina in place. Weaknesses in the pigment epithelium can lead to a detachment of the retina. The retinal pigment epithelium absorbs unwanted light energy from the sclera, cuts down on light scattering, and helps to increase the resolution of our sight. It is also involved with the removal of waste products that accumulate during vision. The rods and cones regularly shed membranes. This shedding occurs in a daily rhythm. The rods shed discs at dawn and the cones shed at dusk. This process may be impaired by genetic defects, drugs or dietary deficiencies. Each retinal pigment epithelial cell must engulf and destroy 2,000 to 3,000 of these disc segments per day or about 90 million discs over an average life span of 80 years!

The retinal pigment epithelium is involved with the metabolism, transport and storage of vitamin A. Vitamin A is an essential component of the visual pigment rhodopsin. Rhodopsin is located in the outer segment disc of rod receptors and is made up of the protein *opsin* combined with *retinol* (Vitamin A- aldehyde). You can see that Vitamin A is a key chemical in the visual pathway, and that a deficiency of this vitamin will have a profound effect on sight. The retinal pigment epithelium is also responsible for the transport and metabolism of two key amino acids that are necessary for retinal function: taurine and methionine

The macula or fovea refers to a small area in the center of the retina, approximately 1.5mm in diameter or about 1/10 of an inch. The foveola is an area of specialized tissue located in the center of the fovea. It contains specialized cones used only for the sharpest of detailed vision. This small area is the location of the earliest changes that take place in ARMD.

Diagnosing Retinal Disease

A careful history is important in evaluating any patient with macular degeneration. The doctor will want to know about the earliest visual symptoms and the age of onset of these symptoms. Loss of vision before age 30 may point to a hereditary form of macular degeneration. If this is the case a careful review of family members should be undertaken. The medical history should be studied along with a drug history. Later on we will talk about several diseases and drugs that are associated with macular degeneration. A careful discussion of the current limitations experienced by the patient should also be reviewed along with realistic goals for the treatment. Since I strongly believe in the effectiveness of good nutrition, I ask my patients about their diets. Most patients need to change their diet and need to begin taking dietary supplements. Other aspects of lifestyle, such as stress management and exercise need to be also examined.

Following the careful history, most eye doctors go through a series of specific tests designed to ascertain a diagnosis of the type of eye disease as well as to determine how the stage of progress of the disease. If you have been to an ophthalmologist, these tests will seem familiar to you. If you suspect to have an eye disease, perhaps knowing what to expect will encourage you for a visit with an eye doctor.

Visual Acuity Testing

It is important to test the near and distance vision in normal lighting conditions. Since this produces some anxiety in patients, I like to put the patient at ease and allow time to read the smallest line possible. Often patients become nervous or uncomfortable during this part of the examination, but it is very important that a base line vision be established before beginning any treatment. I always use a hand held chart and vary the distance from 2 to 5 feet so the patient can read the letters while the doctor records the vision. I also like to note the lighting conditions as well as the time of day the test was given.

In the FDA study that MicroStim Technology Incorporated has initiated, we are using a special chart called, ETDRS, developed by VIH for evaluating dialetic retinopathy. This test uses standardized lighting and will permit us to be even more exact in our evaluation, even when done in many different states.

Color Vision Testing

Testing color vision is also important since a loss of color vision is often part of any disease of the macula. I use either the Ishihara plates or the Farnsworth Hue test. The Ishihara plates are simple and quick, but are more significant when diagnosing color blindness. The patient is asked to read the numbers on 13 color plates. The Farnsworth Hue test is more labor intensive. The patient examines 100 colored bottles and arranges them in order of their colors. Both of these tests are valuable in evaluating the extent of color vision lost and recording progress with treatment.

Amsler Grid Testing

The Amsler Grid is a test used to map the areas of visual loss in the central area of vision. It is a chart with lines that resemble graph paper. Each eye is tested separately. With one eye covered, the patient looks at the center of the paper. Any missing or distorted lines will be noted. This record will be used as a comparison, in the future visits, to note progress in the disease. Patients can also use this tool at home for a more frequent assessment of their progress.

What is Macular Degeneration?

Examining The Front Of The Eye

During this part of the evaluation, the doctor will examine the health of the front part of the eye. He will measure the pressure of the eye to see if there are any signs of glaucoma. He will also evaluate the eye for any signs of a cataract in the lens, which could be reducing the vision

Ophthalmoscopy

This is when the doctor uses a specialized light to look inside the eye. It consists of a specialized light and a series of lenses. This is the part of the examination were the retina and macula are viewed for signs of macular degeneration. The doctor will carefully note any changes and often he will sketch his findings on a piece of paper.

Fluorescein Angiogram

This is a specialized test to study the blood circulation of the retina. The photographs will reveal details of the retinal circulation and also show areas of retinal damage in macular degeneration. It is a painless test where a small amount of dye is injected into the blood stream and a series of photographs the retina are taken from. Small tourniquet is placed on the forearm and a small amount of water-soluble dye is injected into a vein in the arm. This circulates through the bloodstream, including the blood vessels of the eye. In examining these, the doctor is looking for weakness of arteries and possible leakage.

16

This test is usually performed in the office with little discomfort. The dye contains no iodine. A patient can expect his or her skin and urine to be orange-tinged for about half a day. This test is especially useful in evaluating the wet type of macular degeneration. I will discuss more about the types of macular degeneration later in the chapter.

Visual Field Testing

This is a test to measure the peripheral vision. You will be asked to look inside a large white screen the size of a large fish bowl. While looking at the center you will be asked to press a button every time you see a light in your peripheral vision. This test is also important as a baseline to measure your progress with treatment.

Macular Degeneration

What the doctor is looking for is one of a number of diseases that affect the retina and macula. One broad category includes the two types of macular degeneration that affect older persons: Wet and Dry macular degeneration. We call this disease Age-Related Macular Degeneration, or ARMD. Another broad category of diseases is called Hereditary Macular Degeneration. Then there are additional types of macular degeneration related to drug use and other health conditions. I will review all of them in this chapter. All types of macular degeneration can be treated with Microcurrent Stimulation.

Macular Degeneration affects 13 million Americans.

What is Macular Degeneration?

Most of them are over the age of 65, but certain hereditary conditions may cause it to develop in younger individuals. Persons over the age of 75 have a 30% chance of
developing ARMD; it rarely affects anyone younger than
55 years old. It's more prevelant in Caucasians than persons of color because Caucasians have less pigment in
the retina, especially if they have blue, gray, or green eyes.
It affects men and women equally. People who are nearsighted (myopic) have a greater chance of developing the
condition as do people who work or spend a lot of time
out of doors and are exposed to ultraviolet radiation from
sunlight.

What Causes Macular Degeneration?

Macular diseases that are hereditary appear to be
caused by defective genes that somehow impair the development or the functioning of the retina and macula.
There is evidence that these genes impair metalolism of
ATP, the very molecle that MCS seems to enhance. Age-
Related Macular Degeneration (ARMD) is, according to
medical science, a disease of aging and has no specific
cause. Sometimes the symptoms are discussed as causes.
For example, the accumulation of drusen in the retinal
area is said to cause ARMD. But what causes that accumulation? Symptoms are not causes. The cause is more
fundamental than than the accumulation of drussen.

When you examine the relationship between age
and the onset of ARMD, perhaps you will conclude, as I
have, that the same things which afflict so many elderly

are somehow linked to ARMD. These include arthritis, diabetes, hypertension, diseases of the blood vessels, like hardening of the arteries, obesity and high cholesterol. Most of these conditions result from our lifestyle — poor diet, lack of exercise, and the inability to cope with stress. The good news is that things that are caused by factors that we can identify, are more likely to improve when we eliminate those factors. Actually, I believe every disease and disorder has a cause, even childhood cancers. There is no effect without a cause. It would violate the laws of thermodynamics. Medical science likes to say that thing cannot be explained, just because conventional medical science cannot explain them. The truth is they cannot be explained within the framework of demonstrated cause and effect thinking and understanding. Not too long ago, doctors scoffed at the idea that diet had anything to do with heart disease. Until Dr. Dean Ornish proved, within the framework of scientific research, that an improved diet, and a program of exercise, and social support along with relaxation helped reverse physical degeneration, it was impossible to convince doctors of this link. Now that it has been established, however, the medical community has accepted this idea, and lifestyle recommendations are the norm, not just for people with heart disease, but for everyone. We all know that eating less fat and sugar and exercising more are good for us. Coincidentally these same recommendations have been shown to help with diabetes, arthritis, and all the other chronic degenerative conditions that affect our aging population.

What is Macular Degeneration?

In ARMD, vision in the center of the visual field gets fainter and fainter until finally there is hardly any way to see things straight on. The fact that this is a slow process, that it affects older persons, and that it continues to get worse if nothing is done to change the person's lifestyle, leads me to believe firmly that the same factors that produce all degenerative changes in the body are involved in ARMD.

Studies have shown that there is a higher incidence of ARMD in persons who have hypertension, diabetes, and conditions which cause clogging or hardening of the arteries. Therefore, if we can halt or reverse the damage done to our blood vessels and joints through adopting a healthier lifestyle, we can expect improvement in eye conditions like ARMD. This is not just theory; I have seen it work with my patients and so have a number of other ophthalmologists. An added bonus is that the lifestyle recommendations for ARMD are bound to improve other degenerative conditions that patients may have.

If we are going to take a new approach to healing macular degeneration, it is important to take an equally radical view of its cause. Reflect, for a moment, on your own approach to health maintenance and to implementing the lifestyle habits that are known to preserve health. Please do this without guilt. No one is perfect in this regard. We all know enough about nutrition to realize the value of eating five to six servings of vegetables and fruit daily, exercising aerobically several times a week, and using some form of focused relaxation technique daily. It goes without saying that smoking and using alcohol to excess are taboo. Sugar has been implicated in health deterioration in many studies that have been well reported to the public. How do you rate in terms of taking care of yourself. Do you think there might actually be a cause for the degenerative condition that has affected your eyes? If so, are you willing to try to eliminate the cause and adopt techniques and healing methods that might restore your vision?

Microcurrent Stimulation will be far more successful when it is combined with an overall healthy lifestyle. It is a wholistic approach, meaning it effects the whole body. Most of the treatments of conventional medicine 'target' specific, isolated parts of the body. For example, antibiotics target germs, and surgery targets tissue. Holistic or natural approaches to healing, like Microcurrent Stimulation, work synergistically with many aspects of the mind and body. We will talk more about the role of good nutrition in supporting the effectiveness of Microcurrent Stimulation in Chapter Nine. For now, it is enough to understand that the degenerative aspect of Age-Related Macular Degeneration must be addressed and reversed in order for other therapies, including Microcurrent Stimulation, to work optimally. My book, *Healing the Eye the Natural Way: Alternative Medicine and Macular Degeneration,* is an essential reference for anyone who wants to maximize their chances of reversing this disease.

Early Warning Signs of ARMD

Long before vision deteriorates seriously, most people have some warning that their eyes are functioning less effectively. These signs include blurred vision when doing close work, seeing straight lines as wavy, and less intense color vision. Many people notice a lessening of their sight as they look straight at things, like newsprint or faces.. This may be a dimming, a blurring, or actual 'holes' in the vision. In many cases, extreme sensitivity to light and poor night vision also precede ARMD. Light-to-dark adaptation is apt to be very slow. Because other eye conditions may manifest with these same symptoms, it is a good idea to be checked by a qualified eye care professional as soon as you are aware of any signs of vision deterioration.

ARMD rarely leads to total blindness. Instead, worsening symptoms include a loss of central vision and a diminished ability to see things straight ahead. Reading a clock or recognizing a face becomes more and more difficult. People with ARMD come to rely more and more on their peripheral vision. Sometimes, in the early stages, there are holes in vision, (scotomas) or areas where you cannot see anything. Most people with ARMD are declared legally blind and become unable to drive eventually.

Because doctors do not think that anything can be done to halt the progress of this disease, the public has not been educated to be aware of these early symptoms. However, I believe that if people who notice any of these changes in their vision begin to take steps to reverse them, they may be able to arrest the damage to their eyes and maintain normal or near normal vision. ARMD, like most degenerative processes, takes a long time to develop. People may feel that it came on suddenly, but that is because one day they were fine and the next day they received a diagnosis where they feared they may go blind. It does not happen that way. ARMD is a slow progressive disease that may develop for years before it presents any symptoms. Anyone who has been told by their ophthalmologist that they have any of these symptoms would do well to begin using Microcurrent Stimulation immediately to reverse their disease and maintain the highest possible level of eye health. Consider when you are in a movie theatre, at first you are not sure of the dimming. Yet, this dimming is hundreds of times faster than the gradual dimming caused by ARMD.

Wet and Dry Macular Degeneration

ARMD, although one condition in its effects, actually has two types: the wet type and the dry type. These terms have nothing to do with how dry or teary the eyes feel. It refers to two different causes for the macula's deterioration. A person may start with ARMD in only one eye, or have Dry ARMD in one eye and Wet ARMD in the other. This situation will often progress to similar involvement of both eyes.

Wet ARMD occurs when the blood vessels in the back of the eye begin to leak fluid or blood in the back portion of your inner eye. It affects 10% of persons with ARMD. Wet ARMD progresses faster than Dry ARMD and may result in greater loss of vision over a shorter time period. Wet Macular Degeneration has certain characteristics and prognosis (expected outcome). It is possible for Wet ARMD to come on suddenly after a period of stress or shock, and a person may lose a great deal of vision in a short period of time. There are several laser surgical techniques for treating wet ARMD. They tend to preserve vision in the long run, but, because healthy tissue is almost always destroyed along with the diseased vessels, there will often be a short term loss of vision

Dry ARMD, which affects the vast majority of persons with ARMD results from a buildup of cellular waste products in the back part of the eye. These deposits of waste material are called drusen from the German word *druse* meaning bump or gland. Typically a bump develops on Bruch's membrane when the retinal pigment epithelium becomes overloaded with undigested discs from the cones. This collection of waste material produces thickened areas, which look like little bumps or warts. In addition when the *retinal Pigment epithelium* becomes overloaded, these cells begin to degenerate, and debris accumulates at the base of these cells. Fluid begins to accumulate under the cells and soon there are breaks in Bruch's membrane leading to growth and leakage of blood vessels from the choroid. This leakage and new blood vessel growth into the retina lead to the wet stage of macular degeneration. Although we have presented them as seperate conditions, the dry and wet type can be further divided into three characteristic stages, which occur during most types of age-related macular degeneration. Although each situation is unique, there are stages of ARMD that can help you and your doctor determine how advanced your disease is. These stages are important because treatments have been designed based on the stage of your ARMD. Dry ARMD often, but not always, precedes Wet ARMD. When it does precede it, the sequence is as follows:

Dry Stage of Macular Degeneration
1) Development of Drusen
2) Degeneration of Retinal Pigment Epithelial cells
3) Breaks in Bruch's membrane leading to growth and leakage of blood vessels

Wet Stage of Macular Degeneration
The macula is actually the center of the retina. That is why, even when it degenerates, peripheral vision is maintained from images made on the outer circle of the retina. As dead cells build up on the macula, they do two things: they block the macula's ability to produce images and they corrode the delicate tissue, leading to permanent degeneration. It is not certain exactly why the dead cells begin to build up and the 'clean up' mechanism that worked for sixty or more years starts to malfunction, although there is a theory which has been proposed by Dr. Joel Rossen.

What is Macular Degeneration?

As we age, a molecule called ATP, which is abundant in all of our cells, begins to disappear. This particular molecule performs many functions. ATP is a molecule which stores and releases energy in all of our cells, similar to a battery. One of the most important functions of ATP is providing energy to the systems which deliver food to cells and remove metabolic waste. ATP fuels the cellular garbage trucks. When ATP concentrations in the cells are reduced, the cell's ability to rid itself of metabolic waste products, the RPE disks included, becomes greatly compromised. That is when the cellular garbage starts to build up and drusen begins to form. A study done in Belgium a number of years ago proved that MicroCurrent Stimulation increases the ATP in the cells. It also proved that MCS enhanced the cells' abilities to heal themselves and to rid themselves of waste products. This may be one of the reasons MCS is very effective for the treatment of ARMD. Dr. Rossen's theories are presented in greater detail in chapter five.

I have a strong suspicion that the loss of ATP concentration in the cells is very closely related to the process of aging. This means that, as we age, metabolic waste products begin to clog our system and new cells do not regenerate quickly enough to cope with this detritus. The reason this affects the macula so profoundly is that the macula is a very small, highly sensitive area, that is prone to accumulate waste by virtue of its massive metabolic needs.

It is important to recognize that, while this process

occurs over many years, it may not produce any symptoms for a long time. There is no question that Microcurrent Stimulation is most effective when it is used when the condition is less advanced. That is why I urge people over the age of fifty to get regular eye exams, especially now that we know there is something they can do about macular degeneration.

Hereditary Macular Degeneration

There are many types of hereditary retinal degeneration and it would be impossible to discuss them all, but I would like to discuss two types that have responded very well to MCS.

Retinitis Pigmentosa (RP)

In some ways, RP is the opposite of ARMD. While macular degeneration affects only the central vision, RP affects only the peripheral vision. The loss of visual field progresses from the outermost parts of the visual fields toward the center. First the peripheral component of the retina loses function, and the visual loss progress towards the macula. RP is often called progressive tunnel vision, because the patients sees the world through a circle of central vision which becomes smaller and smaller over time.

Retinitis Pigmentosa is a congenital condition that often shows up early in life, but may progress over a longer period of time, even up to forty years. The disorder in the eye, in retinitis pigmentosa is focused on the retina, specifically on the layer of pigment cells beneath the retina. The visual result of retinitis pigmentosa is a constriction of the visual field, with a loss of peripheral vision and a retention of central vision. This is just the opposite of Age-related Macular Degeneration. The changes first begin as a decrease in peripheral vision and a noticeable decrease in night vision. These changes ultimately involve the central area of the retina with loss of central vision. There are variations in the progress of retinitis pigmentosa. Some cases progress very quickly to blindness and others progress slowly.

An important test used in retinitis pigmentosa is the electroretinogram, (ERG). This is a test which measures the response of the retina to light. The ERG can be used to identify the type of retinitis pigmentosa and also to differentiate it from non-genetic retinal disorders. Since RP has several different hereditary patterns, the ERG can be helpful with genetic counseling.

Stargardt's Disease or Juvenile Macular Degeneration

This is an autosomal recessive inherited condition which develops between 6 and 20 years of age. Autosomal recessive means that both parents must carry the trait for the disease, although neither will have it. In Stargard's Disease there is atrophy of the retinal pigment epithelium along with loss of the choroidal circulation. The exact mechanism of visual loss is not known, but evidence points to an early abnormality of the retinal pigment epithelium. Despite the severity of the disease, it has shown consistent positive response to Microcurrent Stimulation.

> James Buchman, one of my patients who has Stargard's Macular Degeneration, was told by his former doctor to go home and wait for blindness to set in — and to be grateful that it might take five years. His wife Robin writes: " James could not believe that he might not be able to see our children grow, watch sunset, enjoy painting, and, still more frightening, lose his job as a teacher, jeopardizing the family's economic situation. I searched the internet and finally found out about your practice, Dr. Kondrot, and MicroCurrent Stimulation. We thank you for giving us hope. Perhaps James will now be able to see his children grow, maintain an active sight-filled life, and pursue his career desires. Without your help we would be preparing for a seeing-eye dog, Braille, and similar life changes."

> Ken Johnson, who tells David's story more completely in Chapter Four, writes this about his son David, another of my patients: "Two and a half months after receiving Microcurrent Stimulation (MCS) at your

office, David. is signing up for college courses. He is talking about driving. Your continuing quest to seek answers when others have quit has changed my son's life. He is now hopeful and optimistic. He is safer and life is easier for him. My wife and I cannot thank you enough.

Macular Degeneration in Diabetes

Diabetes can lead to changes in the retina which cause a decrease in vision. This is due to an increased leakage of retinal blood vessels. There are two areas where this leakage can develop-the space between the cells of blood vessels and the space between the retinal pigment epithelial cells. In some cases of diabetes, small blood vessels will grow into the retina. These blood vessels are very fragile and have a tendency to bleed. This bleeding can cause a loss of vision and the formation of scar tissue. Laser surgery can be very useful in destroying these blood vessels before the complications associated with bleeding develop. Microcurrent Stimulation can help with this condition, but it is not clear whether it can prevent it.

Macular Degeneration with Vascular Disease

Arteriosclerosis can also occur in the retina. Narrowing of blood vessels and blockage of blood vessels can cause the retina not to function. The retina is a specialized tissue which needs a large amount of blood flow, oxygen and nutrients. Any decrease in this supply will make the eye more susceptible to changes associated with macular degeneration

Inflammatory Degeneration

Ocular Histoplasmosis and Ocular Toxoplasmosis are two examples of infectious diseases which can cause degeneration of the macula . These diseases produce inflammation in the eye with changes in the retina and retinal epithelial cells.

Drug-induced Macular Degeneration

Chloroquine, Phenothiazine, Thiordazine are drugs which can produce retinal changes and loss of vision. These drugs appear to accumulate in the retinal pigment epithelium and cause these retinal cells to lose their ability to function properly. Chloroquine is a medication that is commonly used in the treatment of rheumatoid arthritis. Studies have shown that toxicity is related to total dosage of the medication. Patients with a total dose greater than 300 grams per year are at risk. Doctors who prescribe this medication should be aware of this risk and should advise their patients to have a baseline examination before starting this medication. Patients should then have an eye examination every six months while they are taking Chloroquine. The other two medications are less commonly used.

Macular Degeneration Related To Stress

Central Serous Retinopathy is a condition which develops when there is a small area of leakage under the retina which causes a detachment of the macula and a loss of central vision. This condition usually occurs in young men in their 30s or 40s who have a history of great stress followed by a sudden loss of vision. The condition usually resolves over a period of three to six months, but in some cases the retina will have areas of damage with some loss of vision.

The Power of Microcurrent Stimulation

Once we understand the degenerative aspect of Macular Degeneration we can appreciate the power of a treatment that halts the degeneration and reverses the damage already done. Studies in aging have identified several key elements of any attempt to reverse degenerative processes. They are:

1. Increase oxygenation of tissues.
2. Enhance metabolic efficiency.
3. Provide targeted nourishment to tissues and cells.
4. Detoxify tissues and cells.

Fortunately all four of these elements are provided by Microcurrent Stimulation. When you use this phenomenal approach to healing your vision, you will provide all four benefits to your eyes.

Macular Degeneration is a condition that covers a number of specific diagnoses. You are probably reading this book in the hopes that Microcurrent Stimulation can help your condition or that of a loved one. I sincerely hope that is the case. You can find comfort in the fact that my colleagues and I have seen cases of macular degeneration respond to Microcurrent Stimulation and improve at all stages of development. We have also seen that this technique help people of all ages, from young people with hereditary macular degeneration and other retinal problems to folks well into their eighties who have the age-related macular degeneration or ARMD.

What is Macular Degeneration?

2 Why Doesn't my Eye Doctor Know about MCS?

As a nation, we have been taught to trust our doctors. And we do. Many people view doctors as powerful, all-knowing individuals, whose vast experience and extensive training equip them to deal with life and death matters. Our medical system works more efficiently when people do not ask too many questions or request tests and services that lie outside the domain of conventional medicine. Doctors are also rewarded for practicing within what is called the standard of care, or the set of acceptable protocols for treatment. They are rewarded through the trust and approval of their colleagues, by being welcomed into medical societies and groups, and receiving referrals from other doctors. If they practice within managed care, their scope of practice is fairly well determined by the business needs of the organization; in fact they can be censured, demoted, or fired if they do not adhere to the principles of practice set forth within the HMO.

This reality is far from the illusion many patients have of their doctor as a scientist with an open and inquiring mind, eager to learn all about the latest advances in science. This is not to say that doctors do not want the very best for their patients. By and large they do, but they have been trained to believe that the best is synonymous with the status quo until proven otherwise. You may be very surprised to learn that history reveals that it takes at least 50 years for a major new idea, no matter how useful or helpful it is to patients, to become accepted in medical practice. I will discuss some of these facts later in this chapter.

All eye doctors in practice today were told that macular degeneration is a progressive, mostly untreatable, and, certainly, incurable condition, and that nothing can restore a damaged retina to a healthier state. One of the patients who had significant vision improvement as a result of her work with Grace Halloran (see Chapter 3) was told by her doctor: "You can't have gotten better."

Word about Microcurrent Stimulation has been slow to filter throughout the medical community in part because doctors are trained to use only certain sources for information on new procedures and techniques. Treatment approaches, although limited, have focused primarily on wet macular degeneration, a condition caused by fluid leaking into the macula. These techniques have included laser surgery and more recently Photodynamic laser therapy. While reading this book you may find yourself asking, if MCS is such a miracle, why dosen't your eye doctor know about it? The answer to that is very complex, but it does not mean that your doctor is not up to date nor does it infer that MCS is ineffective or harmful.

36

Let's take a look at the history of medicine and see how difficult it is for new treatments to be accepted. One good place to begin is with the story of scurvy and the British navy. Scurvy is a condition that results from the deficiency of Vitamin C and leads to permanent bone malformation and rotting gums. The amount of Vitamin C needed to prevent scurvy is about 60 milligrams. Most people are able to meet their daily needs for Vitamin C through eating enough foods that contain it. However, before refrigeration, sailors on long journeys ate a diet where foods containing Vitamin C were virtually absent. As a result they developed scurvy in large numbers; in fact more died of scurvy than all other diseases and disasters combined.

Around 1750, James Lind, a physician and former sailor conducted a simple test during one single voyage at sea. He gave several small groups of sailors different diets. The ones who received limes and oranges daily quickly recovered from their illness and were able to nurse other sailors. Unbelievable as it seems, it took the British Navy four decades before it allowed limes to be provided to sailors at sea. To this day, English sailors are often called limeys. It was not until 1812 that the practice was mandated. Sixty years were wasted while medical 'scientists' attempted to put aside their conviction that scurvy was contagious or, at least it resulted from evil influences and depression. It was not until 1927 that Vitamin C was discovered.

Another interesting example is the practice of hand

washing to prevent the introduction or spread of germs. Before the widespread use of the microscope, the existence of microbial organisms was not well established. Physicians routinely attended to women in labor or who had just given birth, without washing their hands. Many women, about 10% in fact, developed acute infections known as childbed fever and died shortly after giving birth. One forward looking individual, Ignatz Phillip Semmelweis, observed that the nearby midwife unit had a much lower mortality rate. Due to the loss of his physician friend from infection following a wound inflicted by a knife during an autopsy, Sammelweis concluded that cadaver germs transferred to new mothers caused the problem. He insisted that all the medical students on his ward wash their hands, and his infection rate declined to 1.5%. However, it took twenty years for doctors to adopt this practice, not before they castigated and hounded Semmelweid into a deep depression.

You may be surprised to learn that the tomato was once shunned as food in the belief that it was highly poisonous. Did you know that William Harvey was ostracized from medical circles for saying that blood circulates? Another alarming thing to know is that open-heart surgery was never subjected to research. Once the technology was in place, it very quickly became the standard of practice for certain forms of heart disease. Only later, with retrospective evaluation of cases, did doctors begin to realize that medical management and less invasive procedures produced equally good or better results without the trauma and complications of open-heart surgery. The list goes on, and it must include Linus Pauling whose exhaustive work on Vitamin C received a Nobel Prize in science but whose conclusions regarding the efficacy of Vitamin C are still largely ignored in medical circles. The first patient treated patient treated for retinal degeneration with microcurrent, was treated over 20 years ago.

No discussion of medical science is complete without mentioning the double blind study. When you mention MCS to your doctor, he or she is likely to ask about studies, particularly long-term double blind studies. Doctors have been trained to believe that this is the only way to prove the effectiveness of a new treatment. (Never mind that many drugs are being forced into the marketplace without these studies.) Simply explained, a double blind study means that neither the doctor nor the patient knows which treatment the patient has received. The need for the doctor to be 'blind' is to ensure that he or she does not influence the patient in any way. This is to prevent the 'placebo effect', where people improve just because their doctor suggested they would. In another field this would be called hypnotic suggestion, and might be employed as a powerful and painless way to bring about a desired result. But because medicine is built on the belief of 'standardization', things like personal influence are seen as unacceptable for research. You can see that the double blind model has been developed to test drugs. Very few surgical procedures are subjected to double blind studies because at least half the people would need to be cut open and sewed up without manipulation! MCS is not a treatment that lends itself easily to a double blind approach. Dr. Rossen has recently developed a technique for treating MCS with a double blind study for treatments of ARMD. By the time this book reaches you, FDA clinical trials using Dr. Rossens new techniques may already be under way.

The other form of research, that doctors might accept, is outcome studies. This means that people took the treatment, and had results which was measured outside of changes that might be attributed to anything else. This is the kind of research that MCS is adapted to, and the kind that has been done. These studies have been published, although not in the ophthalmologic journals. Even when MCS is brought to the attention of eye doctors, there may be a lag in its being accepted.

Changes in medicine occur slowly, and the field of ophthalmology has its own story to tell about slow adaptation. The acceptance of the surgical implanting of an intraocular lens is a good example. Cataract surgery involves the removal of the clouded lens from the eye. It is probably the most common intra ocular procedure preformed in the United States. Prior to the insertion of a lens implant, thick cataract glasses were needed to visually rehabilitate the eye after surgery. You may even remember a time when everyone who had their cataracts removed, wore thick glasses for the rest of their lives. These glasses caused many problems such as magnification of central vision, loss of peripheral vision, and loss of depth perception. In many cases the post-operative problems were worse than the visual problems caused by the cataract! The intra-ocular lens was truly remarkable because it eliminated these problems and enabled patients to regain good functional vision. You would expect that eye surgeons were elated when the concept became a possibility.

It is now a routine procedure to insert a lens during cataract surgery although the history of the lens implant is full of controversy. Harold Ridley implanted the first intraocular lens in England in 1949. The reason he experimented with it was due to astute observation of a medical student. During cataract surgery the student asked Dr. Ridley why he did not finish the operation with the insertion of an artificial lens. Ridley had observed many British fighter pilots with plastic shrapnel imbedded in the eye. He also noted that this plastic did not cause damage to the eye. He was open to considering that maybe the medical student had a great idea! He designed a lens implant to help the patient regain natural vision! It wasn't until 3 years later that Warren Reuse MD of Philadelphia performed the first lens implant in the United States.

When this was first introduced, most ophthalmologists called the lens implant a "Time Bomb." The lens was condemned at meetings and comments were made about surgeons massacring the eye. If it wasn't for the efforts of a few visionary eye surgeons who persisted, this wonderful advancement in eye surgery would never have been a part of our life. It wasn't until the late 1970's, more than twenty years later, that intra-ocular lens surgery became an accepted standard in cataract surgery. Why did it take 25 years for this technology to be accepted? Why did so many eye doctors not know about this procedure?

The same thing is happening with microcurrent therapy. Already established in Russia and China as an effective means to treat macular degeneration, it is just beginning to surface in the United States. If history is any predictor most eye doctors will not accept the preliminary results of this exciting technology, despite the fact that there is no other effective treatment for macular degeneration, and there are virtually no side effects. The therapy represents a different paradigm, one that is radically different from surgery and drugs. It uses electricity. I hope it does not take another 25 years, like which occurred with the lens implant, it has been 20 already.

MicroCurrent Stimulation is a relatively new procedure for the treatment of the eye. Currently, only five medical doctors, including myself, have been involved with a preliminary study using MCS in the treatment of macular degeneration. Although the results of MCS in the treatment of wound and pain have been published in many journals, most eye doctors do not have the time to read about studies outside their field. These studies have been available to the medical community, but doctors are very slow to incorporate new information unless it involves surgery or drugs.

Most eye doctors rely on formal, large-scale scientific studies and the publication of results in journals.

Unfortunately these studies take many years to conduct and require even more time to be published. Large studies are expensive to conduct and analyze, and drug companies often underwrite these expenses. For Microcurrent Stimulation there is no such benefactor. Dr. Rossen's company is very small. Inquiries from those interested in supporting his research or investing in his company would be warmly received. I have also explained why it does not lend itself to certain types of research. This does not in the least diminish its effectiveness, however.

Where patients have been treated with Microcurrent Stimulation, all the testing centers have reported positive results with from 60 to 80 percent of patients treated, experiencing an improvement of vision. Dr. Rossen's study is merely underway and it is hoped that the preliminary results of these trials will be available by the end of this year. I hope that this book, *Microcurrent Stimulation: Miracle Eye Cure* and my first book, *Healing the Eye the Natural Way: Alternative Medicine and Macular Degeneration,* will educate eye doctors to recommend this treatment to individuals suffering with macular degeneration. Because there is no harmful aspect to the treatment, and there is no viable alternative to this treatment, I cannot think of a good reason to withhold this option pending the results of long-term studies.

MicroStim® Technology Incorporated, Dr. Rossen's current company, has initiated two clinical trials under the auspices and approval of the Eastern Electromedical IRB (Institutional Review Board) and the

FDA. One trial is evaluating the effects of the MicroStim®
devices on the treatment of dry (non exudative) Age-Related Macular Degeneration (ARMD). The second study
is evaluating the device's effects on a variety of retinal
pathologies including Stargardt's Disease, and both the
wet and dry forms of ARMD. The studies are being done
as part of an ongoing dialogue between MicroStim ® and
the FDA. I am pleased to be one of the primary investigators of these trials. Meanwhile, I continue to use this approach to restore hope and sight for my patients and to
spread the word about this method in every possible way.

My Clinical Experience with MCS

I have been using the MicroStim® 400 and the
MicroStim® 100 microcurrent stimulators in my practice
since August of 1998 and have been very impressed with
the improvements I have seen in the vision of patients
with macular degeneration. Most of my patients begin to
see an improvement after four days of treatment, even if
they have suffered deteriorating eyesight for years! Read
some of their stories in Chapter 4. Take their stories as
motivation for yourself. Read on to learn how to use MCS
at home. Call me to obtain a unit and get started on improving your vision.

3	**There is Hope. The Story of Grace Halloran and Her Work.**

I want to introduce you to one of the pioneers in the use of Microcurrent Stimulation in the United States. Dr. Grace Halloran is not only a selfless contributor to the evolving science of treating "incurable" eye conditions with natural methods, she is a wonderful human being. She has worked with hundreds of visually impaired individuals through her program of Intregrated Visual Healing. She conducts week-long sessions in Northern California and draws participants from around the world and the country. Clients who work with her leave with a complete program of home treatments to continue their vision improvement. For thos unable to attend, a workbook and supplies can be ordered from her. More information on the IVH program is provided in the Resources section.

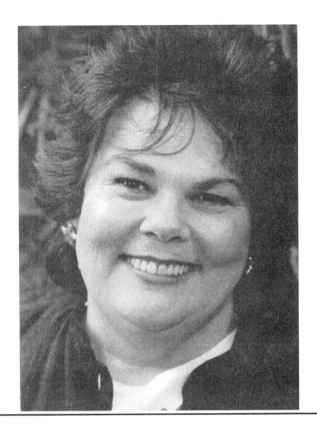

Grace Halloran, Ph.D. Founder,

Intregrated Visual Healing (IVH) Program.

Grace was born into a family where most of the adults developed Retinitis Pigmentosis (RP). Her eyesight began to fail in her twenties, just at a time when she was beginning to redeem what, until then, had been a very difficult and quite self-destructive life. While seeking treatment for her headaches, she learned she had the genetic disorder Retinitis pigmentosis and was already legally blind. Specifically she was diagnosed with Retinitis Pigmentosa and cystoid macular degeneration. She had less than five degrees of field vision in both eyes and less than 20/200 central acuity. She was told she would be completely blind in a few years. "I was told to learn Braille, get a dog, and not even think about a cure." With typical Grace resilience, her response was gratitude that she did not have brain tumor, which she had suspected due to the headaches. Grace's story is told in her wonderfully inspiring and moving book, *Amazing Grace, Autobiography of a Survivor*. (See Resources)

Her book is, in part, the story of her search for a cure for RP and the story of her search for a child she had given up for adoption when she was very young. Her baby daughter had been separated from Grace before she knew about the RP in her family. As the mother of two children, both of whom were highly likely to also develop the disease, she committed her life to finding a treatment for this disease in time to save her children from the same fate. She not only had to find a cure; she had to find her child. Despite a daunting number of difficulties and setbacks in life, her response was always to look on the bright side of events, and to be willing to commit to the healing of others. When asked how she has maintained so much optimism in the face of so many difficulties, Grace answered:

"Why did I not give up like others? In the

beginning, I was determined to help prevent my children from going blind, and had not expected to see any improvement for myself. When I began to see changes for the positive, I became cautiously optimistic. Then, the whole world opened up and I enjoyed good usable, functional vision for many years. Then, on a trip to Europe I suffered from the exposure to the radiation of Russia's Chernobyl nuclear power plan accident, and my health and vision began to deteriorate. In 1993 I lost all my sight, and my thyroid. I did give up. I was overwhelmed and felt that I had no hope for health or sight. What turned me around were other people wanting me to help them fight their own eye disorders. Through their desires, I began to research and experiment with the new technologies and scientific breakthroughs in nutrition and the micro current therapy. Not knowing what I could do for my own sight, I knew it at the very least wouldn't hurt, so I started in earnest. Now I can read the computer screen, see some colors, and best of all, see my grandchildren. I know that there is always room for improvement, and that I will never, ever give up for longer than fifteen minutes."

In 1979, Dr. Grace Halloran, who was then living in Marin County in California, became the first person in the United States to use microcurrent for the treatment of retinal disease. A series of unlikely events led to her involvement, and to her becoming a pioneer in the field of vision healing and training.

At that time she was working as a consultant to the football team at Sonoma State University, in Penngrove, California. Her specialty was the alternative treatment of injuries. Her friend, Dr. Jack Scott, who was a physical therapist and a consultant to the Olympic Ski Team, introduced her to Microcurrent therapy and to his friend, Dr. Joel Rossen. MicroCurrent Stimulation (MCS) had existed for just over one year at that time. Dr. Rossen, a veterinarian, had the distinction of being one of the few people in the world, at that time, who was trained in the technology of Microcurrent stimulation, animal and human acupuncture, and veterinary medicine. He is also the inventor of the MicroStim® technology. Grace purchased an MCS device from Dr. Rossen's company, was trained by Joel and Jack, and she started using Microcurrent with the football team to treat injuries. She worked with Dr.Rossen to refine the frequencies and the selection of the acupuncture points over the course of several years. At that time she did not know where this would lead, but her son, Kevin, helped her chart her course.

The day before his eighth birthday, Kevin broke his elbow. He was roughhousing with one of his friends, and landed hard on his arm. 'Crack' and the elbow was fractured in two places. Off to the hospital they went. After taking X-Rays, the orthopedist told Grace that reduction of the fractures would require surgery. A closed reduction was out of the question. The swelling was too severe to reduce the fractures without cutting. There was serious damage to the growth plates, the swelling was quite severe, and she was told that the arm might not grow any more. Kevin might have an arm the size of an eight-year old for the rest of his life. Surgery (open fracture reduction) was offered as the only solution, and Dr. Halloran consented. Who could have imagined where that would lead?

All the operating rooms were already in use and there was not to be a room available until midnight, sic hours away. Grace was left to wait with her boy who was in incredible pain, with his elbow swollen to the size of a football. Fortunately, she had her Microcurrent Stimulation device with her. She knew how effective it had been with the football team in pain control. So she began treating Kevin's fracture intermittently about half a dozen times over the next six hours. After the second treatment, Kevin reported that his pain had stopped. Every hour, the swelling went down a little more.

At midnight, when the operating room was finally available, Kevin was taken in for his open reduction. He was anesthetized and prepped for surgery. Shortly thereafter, he was returned to Grace. The doctors said that the swelling had subsided so much that the surgical part of the procedure was cancelled, and the fracture was reduced by the closed method.

The next day, Dr. Jack Scott got Kevin a fiberglass cast. Grace and Jack drilled holes in the cast and continued to treat Kevin with Microcurrent Stimulation daily for the next six weeks. The follow-up x-ray at six weeks showed a healing fracture that no longer even required a cast. He was out of the cast in only six weeks. Kevin is now 28 years old and in the Air Force. He stands six feet four inches, and he has a perfectly matched set of strong arms.

After seeing her son heal so beautifully, Grace thought, " Why not try this on my eyes?" She began to treat herself on a daily basis for the next year. During that time, she met periodically with Dr. Rossen, and they collaborated to fine tune the techniques she was using to treat herself. Within one year, Dr. Halloran's vision had improved so much that she passed her driving test, and was qualified for night driving. She bought her first car, a bright, shiny, red pickup truck.

Grace had been working on improving her vision for a number of years prior to the addition of Microcurrent Stimulation to her regime. At one point, she had had an electroretinogram test (ERG) prior to the beginning of her self-help program and the result was a 'flat line.' The ERG is the gold standard for diagnosis of RP, and is objective and conclusive. A flat line ERG is never repeated because the assumption is that there will never be any improvement. Grace says, "After working with the Micro Current I knew my fields were better. I went back to my doctor and had to demand that another ERG be given. The result was that, after a year or two of applying micro current therapy, I had some "peaks and valley's" show up on a new ERG. It was still abnormal, but it was no longer a flat line. That was proof positive that my retinal function had indeed improved. My night vision was much better, my central acuity was improved and my fields expanded as well. Overall, my entire visual function was demonstrably better. Improvements like that do not happen spontaneously in RP."

In her book she expresses her joy at this turn of events. "No one ever appreciated the outdoors and the highways as I did…. With the return of mobility my feelings of appreciation and gratitude brought tears of joy to my eyes. People must have thought we (she and her son) were a tad backwards, singing and laughing as we traveled the byways and back roads into the wilderness."

Grace's happiness was boundless at this juncture in her life. Not only could she see to function normally and freely in life, she felt certain she could prevent her condition from manifesting in her son.

Since then, her dedication to beating degenerative retinal diseases, not only for herself, but also for her children and for everyone afflicted with the problem has never ceased. During the next three years, Grace treated friends and family and worked at four different optometry practices. She achieved consistently good results with most of the RP and ARMD clients that she treated.

Her personal journey brought many challenges as

well as rewards. She was reunited with her daughter, who now works with her in the Integrated Visual Healing seminars. As a result of finding Kathy, two wonderful grandchildren have become part of her life in addition to the child her son eventually had. Grace's health was severely challenged as a result of radiation poisoning during the nuclear accident in Chernobyl, while on a worldwide speaking tour. This permanently damaged her thyroid gland, which was removed back in the states. As a result her vision deteriorated. Despite this tragedy she remains committed to helping others regain their sight.

> To Quote Grace, " My prognosis according to conventional medical doctors is not good. However, in 1993, when I lost all my sight, and went completely blind, I gave up completely. In helping others, I have continued to use my own program of therapies on myself. Now, I am able to read the computer screen, see some colors, and most importantly, see my grandchildren's faces a pure joy."

Intregrated Visual Healing

The Integrated Visual Healing program developed by Grace Halloran, Ph.D. is a-unique and innovative approach to serious eye disorders. As both patient and practitioner, Grace provides an intensive educational and therapy program for people facing sight loss due to serious eye disorders. The IVH program incorporates cutting edge technology in the micro-current stimulation field, utilizing the MicroStim® for home use. Each participant in this intensive training gets personalized instruction and practice using this equipment. The IVH program offers recommendations for three levels of intervention: prevention, maintenance, and therapeutics for eye health recovery. Grace believes that each individual can become his or her own eye health therapist. Over a four-day period, with more than 24 hours of instruction and practice, she provides a specific, step-by-step program for each individual to continue at home.

The IVH program emphasizes nutrition in much the same way that I have in a later chapter in this book. Grace also talks about the importance of good digestion, and eating only high quality unadulterated food.

Other disciplines included in IVH are: color therapy, stress management, eye health exercises, acupressure and Total Body Balancing. Each of these disciplines has been tailored to eye health and visual function. When they are combined, the result is the best possible outcome for eye health improvement and sight recovery. The true success of her program is shown over the years of participants' ongoing vision improvement. These are participants who have eye disorders that are typically on a downhill course with no hope of recovery.

For those who are unable to attend this dynamic and intensive training workshop, Grace has developed home training materials, making this a remarkable self-

help program for anyone facing visual challenges.
Reversing Macular Degeneration Seminars

Grace Halloran and I now conduct two-day workshops around the county for people with macular degeneration and other eye disorders resulting in sight loss. In
these seminars we present information about the various treatments used to reverse macular degeneration.
These seminars combine the unique talents of two individuals who have made the discovery of alternative ways
to heal from vision loss their life's work. Of course,
Microcurrent Stimulation is one of the featured subjects.
Information about Reversing Macular Degeneration
workshops is provided at the end of this chapter.

There is Always Hope

Slowly, the medical and scientific community has
awakened to the benefits of further use, as well as research on Microcurrent. People like Grace Halloran are
the secret benefactors of many. She has kept hope in healing vision alive through years of personal and professional hardship. Every person who has or will benefit
from Microcurrent Stimulation owes her a debt of gratitude. Even more significantly, scientists and doctors who
are now undertaking the new level of investigation into
Microcurrent Stimulation are building on the early work
of an underpaid and unrecognized pioneer. Often the
most profound contribution to any field comes from
someone who is afflicted with the condition under study.
It is rare, though, that this contributor is as loving and

professionally accomplished as Grace Halloran.

Grace and I both know that most people who consult with us and come to our workshops, have been told to abandon hope of regaining their vision. This is her message to people who have been told to give up:

> "Most people want to be fixed by someone else so they don't have to change anything about themselves. That's their path. I know that the path I choose–the journey towards improved sight and health–is a challenging one. For those who want to explore their universe, to find answers that were hidden, I say, 'don't give up. Reach out, ask the questions that need asking, because the answers are always available.' It takes a special type of person to take risks, and I welcome them to my world, a world of hope, optimism and great joy and adventure. There is always hope, and don't ever let anyone tell you differently."

<table>
<tr><td>**4**</td><td>**Patients Tell Their Story**</td></tr>
</table>

You have learned quite a lot about Microcurrent Stimulation already. The next chapter will teach you how to set up and use your unit. Before we get to that, however, I want you to read the stories of some of my patients who have benefited from MCS therapy. Each patient whose story of recovery is told in this chapter, has beaten the odds against macular degeneration. The first two stories, those of Joanne Lew and R.E., talk about recovering a significant amount of vision in persons who have age-related macular degeneration. The last story is the poignant tale of a young boy whose life, and indeed his future, was compromised by his congenital macular disease. This one still brings tears to my eyes, worked for them too.

Today, my son lives on his own; he is safer. He can see things better and can relate better. His eyesight is 90% of what a normal person sees; up from 75%. He has had to re-learn to read, and now does it for pleasure. He is thinking about how to structure the next phase of his life, and going back to school. He is taking the lead in nity. So, read on and let the voices of people like yourself inspire you.

Joanne Lew: An Artist with Macular Degeneration

Joanne Lew's story illustrates the importance of having regular eye check-ups. Her Macular degeneration was detected during a routine visit to my office. Although she had been having some minor visual disturbances that are typical of ARMD, she had no idea that such a potentially serious disease process was underway deep within her eyes. If you wonder about the amazing recovery this woman has made, take a look at the painting she did of her great granddaughter just six months ago. This painting won best of show in the Bethel Artist's Guild's annual, juried exhibit in Pittsburgh in 1999. Joanne is very proud of this award. We have reproduced the painting on the following page. You know that whoever painted this picture of an adorable one-year old was able to see extremely well and had a real eye for color. Read on for Joanne's story, as she tells us that it was not always that way.

Joanne Lew is a registered nurse. She lives in Pittsburgh, Pennsylvania, with her husband, Raymond and stepson, Steven. Joanne is 66 years old, and, although she is young for such an honor, she is the great grandmother of one, grandmother of eight, and mother of four.

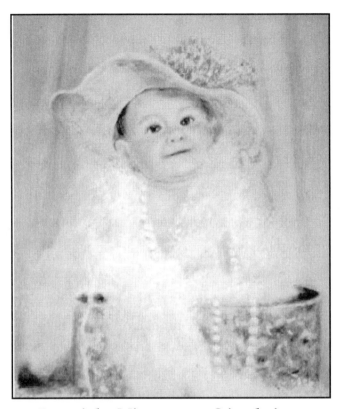

Portrait by Microcurrent Stimulation
Patient, Joanne Lew. Best of Show, 1999
Bethel Artist's Guild

I first met Joanne when, as a private duty nurse, she brought one of her own patients to my office for a consultation. During the visit she asked me to look at an abnormal growth in the corner of her eye. I diagnosed it as a cyst and suggested she have it removed as soon as possible. We set the surgery for later that week. The cyst was benign and she recovered without any problems.

"I began to notice a loss of close vision a

few years later," Joanne says. "The numbers on the face of the alarm clock were impossible for me to see. My color perception was dimming too. I got reading glasses, but had no reason to be concerned. However, when Dr. Kondrot told me, during a routine eye exam, that I had macular degeneration, I was devastated. All I could think of was waking up one day and finding a big hole in my central vision. I knew from my nurse's training that there was no treatment. Naturally, when he suggested that Microcurrent Stimulation might help, I jumped at the chance."

"I laugh when I recall how intimidated I was by using the unit at first. It is so easy to use! But, at first, I thought, 'I'll never be able to do it.' I had a training session in Dr. Kondrot's office several times within a week. He also gave me some very useful literature. I have been on the program, using the unit twice a day, for about a year and a half. It is just part of my life. Using the unit is easy and pleasant. It takes me about 40 minutes each time, including the set up.

Joanne is in generally good health except for a tendency toward high cholesterol levels, "which is now under control," she says, because "I'm eating the cardiac diet recommended for my husband. It is low in fat and cholesterol and high in fiber and fruits and vegetables." She also takes the Macular Degeneration Formula daily. Her goal is to exercise more and, as for stress reduction, she does nothing special, although she alludes to being in a very good phase of life that has had its share of problems. Of course, the joy of her life is having 20/20 vision in her left eye, and nearly 20/20 in her right eye as well as sharp color vision. She attributes the miracle of her nearly perfect sight to regular use of Microcurrent Stimulation for a little over one year.

> "I am less dependent on my reading glasses
> now, which is unusual for someone my age.
> And, the other day I glanced at the alarm
> clock and was able to see the numbers very
> well; they were completely clear."

R.E. – A Senior Who Can Drive Again

R.E., who lives in Connecticut, is 76 years old. After not being able to drive for three months, due to Macular Degeneration, he is back on the road. "Poor eyes run in my family," he says. "My Dad had Macular Degeneration, somewhere in his late seventies." R.E. attributes the miraculous return of his vision to Microcurrent Stimulation, exercise, prayer, and a focus on nutrition, including the herb, Bilberry. He juices vegetables – kale, carrots, broccoli, and cucumbers - and drinks the juice every day. "I was trained as an engineer, and I have designed a program for myself that is bringing results."

R.E. was diagnosed with Macular Degeneration by his local ophthalmologist. He learned about MicroCurrent Stimulation on the internet in an article about Sam Snead's recovery of sight using MCS. This led him to Dr. Khouri in Florida, who showed him how to use the MCS unit.

> "My early symptoms included fog in my central vision, distortions of lines, and some episodes of double vision. I tested at 20/100 on my first visit. After using MCS, I went back to my original ophthalmologist for a check-up less than a year later. I did not tell him about the MCS. 'What have you done?' he asked me in astonishment, as he compared the state of my eyes to photos he had taken on the first visit. 'You've had laser treatment, haven't you?' Actually, Dr. Kondrot said the same thing to me when I finally met him earlier this year, and he had chance to examine me and look at these original photos."

R.E. does MCS four times a week for fifteen minutes each time. He has added the acupressure points found in Grace Halloran's workbook to his routine. Currently, reading is still somewhat of a problem, but he can read with vision aides and good lighting. "This too is clearing up," he says quite happily.

> "Finally, after seventy-six years, I know what it means when people say that God talks to them. I feel that I have been given guidance and opportunities. In, fact, I have made a sort of deal with the Lord. 'You help me see better, and I'll help others see better.' I help others with vision problems through a telephone support group. I try to keep on top of new developments and pass them on. In fact, I've recently had homeopathic treatment from Dr. Kondrot, and I know, definitely, that this is helping me. After two months on homeopathy, I can see the strength coming to my eyes. I may need to do Microcurrent Stimulation for the rest of my life, that is unless my homeopathic treatment is so successful that I can stop or reduce my work with MCS. However, this is no problem as MCS is so easy to do and so effective."

Patients Tell Their Story

Ken Johnson: My Son Has Reclaimed his Life

"When my son, David was ten years old, he began to have trouble seeing the blackboard at school. His teacher suggested we get his eyes checked. Little did I know that this would be the beginning of a nightmare odyssey in the medical world. We consulted several optometrists and ophthalmologists who could not diagnose his eye problems. Finally we went to the Wheaten Clinic where we were told he has Stargardt's disease. This is a juvenile form of macular degeneration that is congenital. As far as we know, no one in my wife's or my family has the disease, but, apparently, we each carry a recessive gene. That gave any of our children a one in four chance of developing the condition. As we were about to learn, a diagnosis of Stargardt's is a sentence to a life of semi-invalidism. Our son was told he would never drive. We soon found out that he had difficulty reading. Therefore, his main activity, going to school, became a huge challenge."

"We were referred to Northwestern Hospital for a more definitive work up. At the conclusion of many tests there, the leading physician told us that she actually questioned the diagnosis. We traveled to Mayo Clinic in the hope of getting some definitive information, and, frankly, still looking for hope."

"At Mayo, we got the news that David definitely had Stargardt's, and that nothing could be done about it. We were told to begin preparing him to adapt to a life without driving and sports, and many of the other things young boys like to do."

"Virtually the only good news was the condition would most likely stabilize at his present visual acuity of 20/200. This could not be corrected. He had very poor central vision, but good peripheral vision. The drive home was terrible; it was the longest trip I can recall. Back home we settled into a mode of acceptance – or tried to anyway. We looked for aids to help David study, but there was nothing he could use in the classroom. We eventually relied on oral instruction for him. He had given up all hope regarding his eyesight, even as he watched his buddies get their drivers' licenses and gain more and more independence. And so, eight precious years passed. David graduated from high school, and we all felt relief that that struggle was over. However, what would become of this young man was still unresolved."

Actually, I had never given up hope. One day, while searching the website I read about a study funded by the Macular Degeneration Association. It involved something called Microcurrent Stimulation. Dr. Edward Kondrot in Pittsburgh was one of three doctors involved. I tried to get more information about this technique but not much was available. Finally I asked David if he would like to give it a try.

In May, of '99, we went to see Dr. Kondrot. Meeting him was an entirely different experience than any we had had, since no one had offered any hope. The other doctors told us there was nothing that could be done now and no prospects for the future. Dr. Kondrot looked me square in the eye and said he would do everything possible for our son.

David received instructions and MCS treatment at Dr. Kondrot's office over a period of four days. After the second treatment, he saw a 'clearing' in his visual field. Things were not as blurry as before. His sight was even better on day three, and then maintained that level on the fourth day. We were told that that is normal.

We returned home with the MCS unit, bottles of Pure Focus, Aldous Huxley's book, *The Art of Seeing*, and a series of eye exercises to do daily. I couldn't help but wonder why no one else, at all the prestigious medical centers, had been able to offer us anything at all.   I have a scientific background and am an executive at a leading health care company, so I am not one to grasp at straws. But the truth was that my son's vision was steadily improving. Perhaps most important, his spirits picked up.

In my enthusiasm I decided to contact Mayo Clinic and tell them about this discovery so that they could offer it to others. They wrote back saying that there is no evidence that Microcurrent Stimulation helps people regain eyesight. No evidence? I had evidence for them, but they were not interested.

We were told to expect improvement over a course of three months. We did the MCS treatments four times per week. When we went back to the Wheaten Clinic to have his eyes re-tested, his sight had improved from 20/200 to somewhere between 20/120 and20/160. There was a marked and distinct difference in what he could see. I was very encouraged, and feel some obligation to spread the word. I financed someone else to have this treatment and it worked for them too.

Today, my son lives on his own; he is safer. He can see things better and can relate better. His eyesight is 90% of what a normal person sees; up from 75%. He has had to re-learn to read, and now does it for pleasure. He is thinking about how to structure the next phase of his life, and going back to school. He is taking the lead in planning his future, as he should be at the age of nineteen. We are not concerned about him any more. Just very grateful. The best thing Dr. Kondrot ever gave us was hope.

5 History of Microcurrent Stimulation

The history of MCS is a long and interesting one. The first report of the use of an electrical current to treat disease is from the Roman physician Scribonius Largus in 46AD. He described using the black torpedo fish to treat gout. This fish would produce an electrical shock when frightened, and Largus advised persons with gout to stand in the surf and step on the fish. The electrical current produced by the fish was reputed to eliminate the terrible pain of gout.

There is some evidence that the ancient Egyptians (2500 BC) also knew of this treatment. Stone carvings of a species of catfish called Malapterurus electrus are found in hieroglyphics. These historical reliefs may be the first 'written' records of electricity being used to treat painful conditions in the same method done in in Rome, using the shock of an electrical fish.

It wasn't until 1745 that a device was developed that could actually store and supply electricity for the treatment of pain. This was first called the Leyden jar. Later, this device became the "Electreat". The device received a US patent in 1919 and sold for $12.50. The Electreat was the precursor of the modern day Transcutaneous Electrical Nerve Stimulation or TENS unit. This device is the prototype of the Microcurrent Stimulation unit.

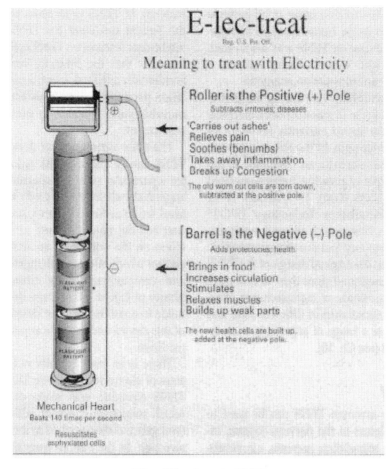

The Electreat, 1919

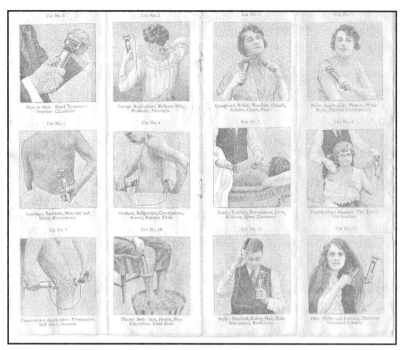

From the Electreat Manual, 1919

How To Treat Yourself

In 1965, two researchers named Melzack and Wall published a book on the gate control theory and dorsal column nerve stimulation. The gate control theory is an explanation of the transmission and treatment of pain. It suggests that there is a gate on the spinal cord which acts as an on or off switch for the transmission of pain. This gate then allows the pain impulse to proceed to the brain or it has the ability to stop the pain.

Let's look at the beginning of the process when a pain fiber is first stimulated. There are pain receptors called nociceptors, which are located all over the skin and

71

body. These nociceptors are activated by a painful stimulus such as heat, pressure, cold or trauma. Once the receptors are stimulated, chemicals are released which stimulate the nerves, which in turn send pain signals to the spinal column. We do not feel pain until these pain impulses travel up the spinal cord to the brain; only then is pain perceived. It is at the dorsal column of the spinal cord that the impulse is then conducted to an area of the brain called the thalamus. The thalamus acts as a relay station for most types of pain sensation.

Melzak and Wall discovered that an electrical stimulus at the dorsal column would prevent the sensation of pain. The dorsal column of the spinal cord is an area on the back of the spinal cord where nerves that conduct pain to the brain are located. This research made possible the development and medical use of the first generation of Transcutaneous Electrical Nerve Stimulators (TENS units) that have helped hundreds and thousands of patients to control pain. Helpful as these were and are, they do little to actually heal the painful site, although they often bring great relief.

It took nearly sixty years before the next big breakthrough in electrical stimulation surfaced. Although no one can really say for sure at this time, it seems that Dr. Thomas Wing may have been the father of the next generation of electrical stimulator, the MicroCurrent Stimulator. Somewhere around the end of the 1970s, Dr. Wing introduced his Acu-O-Matic device.

Although TENS devices are primarily used for the

treatment of pain, a number of other effects have been reported. Several studies have found that using the TENS unit increases blood flow and stimulates wound healing. Kjartansson and Lundeberg in 1990 did a study on 20 patients who had poor skin circulation due to plastic surgery. After using the TENS treatment their skin showed a significant increase in blood flow.

Debreceni in 1995 reported the results in using the TENS unit for circulatory problems. Twenty-four patients were studied who had blockage of the arteries to their lower leg, which resulted in poor circulation and pain. After the TENS treatment, twenty patients showed marked improvement. There was decrease in pain, reduction in pain on walking, and healing of persistent ulcers after the TENS treatment.

Kaada in 1982 studies the effects of TENS in four patients with Raynauds extreme coldness in the hands resulting from constricted blood vessels. Diabetic polyneuropathy is numbness in the extremities, usually the feet, due to nerve damage. Both of these conditions produce symptoms of coldness, numbness, pain, and loss of movement. Results of his study showed that treatment with the TENS unit increased the skin temperature and brought relief to the patients.

The following year in 1983, Kaada studied the effect of TENS in the treatment of chronic leg ulcers. Ten patients treated. These patients had leg ulcers which had resisted the standard medical approaches. After the treatment with TENS, eight of the ten patients had successful healing of their leg ulcers!

We have seen that MCS can be of value in the treatment of circulatory problems and ulcers that do not heal. What is the mechanism of this weak electrical current, when it is applied to the skin and how can it help the disease of macular degeneration? We must look at the smallest part of our body, the cells, to understand the effect of MCS. The cells, as we know are the building blocks of the body, and they must function properly for life, and, in the case of the eye, for vision to occur. An important component of the cell is the mitochondria. Each cell is composed of thousands of mitochondria, which are the source of energy for the cell to function. In order to generate energy, a chemical reaction takes place in the cell in which ATP is required. ATP is the fuel that the mitochondria needs to generate energy. The cells use this energy to convert amino acids into proteins that are used for the functions of life and vision. So there are three things a cell needs: healthy mitochondria, ATP, and the ability to make protein. The following experiment demonstrates how the use of MCS enhances cells' functioning.

In 1982. Ngok Cheng studied the effects of TENS on the skin of the rat. He applied different levels of current on the surface of the rat skin and then studied the changes in the cells using electron microscopy. This technique enabled him to observe the changes in the cellular mechanics. His results indicated that between 50 and 500 microamperes will cause an increase in mitochondria activity and an increase of 300 to 500 percent in ATP levels. He also noted that at this level there was an increase in protein synthesis and gluco-neogenesis. This study is exciting because it gives us a model on how MCS might work inside the eye. The MCS applied to the eye will stimulate the diseased retinal cells, increasing cellular functions and stimulating the diseased cells to recover.

Elsewhere in this book, you have read the story of Dr. Grace Halloran. The work of Dr. Halloran is the seed from which a network of physicians has grown who use the MicroStim® for treatment of retinal degeneration. Several years after Grace's initial discovery of microcurrent's value for treating RP, Dr. Joel Rossen, inventor of the MicroStim®, presented a pain management seminar in San Francisco. An optomotrist from South Dakota, Dr. Leland Michael, attended the seminar, as did Grace. By that time, 1985, Grace was the founder and president of the Center for Eye Health education, in Santa Rosa. Dr. Rossen was on her board.

At Dr. Rossen's seminar, Grace and Dr. Michaels struck up a friendship. Dr. Michaels completed his West coast trip with a visit to Grace's facility to be trained in her procedures for treating RP and ARMD with microcurrent electrical stimulation. That training was the beginning of a study that lasted nearly eight years and consummated with the publication of an article in the Journal of Orthomolecular Medicine in 1993. Dr. Michaels reported the findings on a group of 25 ARMD patients who were followed from 1985 to 1992. The study indluded both wet and dry ARMD patients. Dr. Michaels reported that over the course of the study, there was an average improvement in the vision of 1.4 letters. One patient with the wet type had a severe bleeding which caused a 66 letter loss in that eye. Discounting the extreme skew in the data created by this one patient, there was a 66 letter average improvement in the left eye during the same period. Although it is difficult to separate the data from the wet and dry patients, it is clear that there was a net average gain of visual acuity in both eyes of the patients with dry ARMD. Unfortunately, Dr. Michaels died shortly after completing that phase of the study. His practice was taken over by Dr. John Jarding.

In October 1997, Dr. Rossen attended a Symposium given by the International Association for Biologically Closed Electrical Circuits. Several papers were presented on the treatment of ARMD with microcurrent stimulation. Dr. John Jarding, Dr. Larry Wallace, President and Director of the College of Syntonic Optometry, and Dr. Grace Halloran all presented papers validating rge effectiveness of microcurrent stimulation in the treatment of Macular Degeneration.

At that time, the devices of choice were those manufactured by MicroStim® Technology Incorporated. Dr. Joel Rossen, president of MicroStim, had developed and patented a unique line of microcurrent stimulators. It was at that seminar that Damon Miller MD, decided to purchase MicroStim® and begin treating patients with ARMD as part of his practice. The statistical analysis of

Dr. Millers patients appear elsewhere in this book.

After Dr. Miller, the next four doctors to start using MicroStim® devices for treatment of ARMD were all ophthalmologists. Dr. George Khouri , of West Palm Beach Florida, started in February 1998, Dr. Percival Chee, of Honolulu Hawaii, started in May 1998, I started in August 1998 and then Dr. James Nagel, of Waukesha Wisconsin, started in March of 1999. The Macular Degeneration Center of Colorado Springs opened in April 1999 under the direction of Dr. Joyce Gamewell, herself a Macular Degeneration patient. She chose to open a center for the treatment of degenerative retinal disease because she had regained her sight after a visit to Dr. Miller.

History of MCS

6

Can Microcurrent Stimulation Help You?

As we take you through this remarkable journey of a powerful method for restoring your vision, you may begin to question whether Microcurrent Stimulation can offer any hope for you, personally. You may be someone who has received a diagnosis of macular degeneration and has been told that there is nothing that can be done. You were understandably shocked when the eye doctor told you that you have Macular Degeneration! You felt numb when he told you that stronger glasses would not help and that nothing could be done to improve your vision. "How can this be?" you wondered. "I live a healthy lifestyle and eat the right food. The doctor has made a mistake; perhaps I should get another opinion." Your second opinion confirms the diagnosis of macular degeneration. "Why has this happened to me?" you may protest.

Alternatively, you may be in the beginning stages of changes in your vision that you suspect indicate something serious. Perhaps you may have noticed some changes in your ability to see or to focus. Objects may not be as clear as they once were, and you may have noticed more difficulty with reading. You may also notice that sometimes things are distorted or wavy. "Oh it is time to get a change in my glasses", you tell yourself. Deep down, however, you may suspect something worse, but you do not want to admit it.

Denial is a perfectly normal reaction when a person first receives a diagnosis of macular degeneration, whether the cause is age-related or heredity. Anger, and later, fear are also normal reactions. You may feel singled out for this condition when your friends and spouse are free from it. "Why me?" is a normal feeling. "Why my eyes? I have so much to do in life." Later, perhaps hours or weeks later, when you face the implications of the loss of your sight you might undergo, feelings of fear. "Who will take care of me if I become blind?"

Losing your vision produces the same type of shock as the death of a loved one. After all, your ability to see is one of your best friends in life. It allows you to navigate safely through life and grants you the opportunity to appreciate the beauty of this world. Elizabeth Kubler Ross is a psychiatrist who studied the reactions to loss. She learned that people go through five predictable phases in response to any major loss. She described these in her pioneering work, On Death and Dying, published in 1974.

1. Denial
2. Anger
3. Bargaining
4. Depression
5. Acceptance.

Bargaining refers to our tendency to 'strike a deal' with fate or God in order to be relieved of the burden or disease that has overtaken us. At this stage you might feel tempted to promise to improve your diet or give up an unhealthy substance or exercise in exchange for healthy eyes. Even though you know this is irrational, you may find yourself thinking along these lines.

The stage of Depression is actually, according to Dr. Kubler-Ross, depression exists only if the symptom he called Learned Helplessness is present. Learned Helplessness means that the subject has "learned and accepted" that there is nothin more that can be done. Once the learned helplessness is extinguished, the patient can move on and healing may begin.

Although you have to go through all these stages, I ask you to avoid the last one, acceptance. While you need to accept that your vision now requires your attention in order to improve, there is no need to give up hope for its improvement. For most of you, you no longer need to feel helpless. Microcurrent Stimulation can improve your vision and bring back your precious sight.

Can MCS Help You?

The First Step Is The Eye Examination.

If you are concerned about your eyes, but do not know exactly what is wrong with them, the first step you need to take is to have a thorough eye examination with either an ophthalmologist or an optometrist. There are many causes of decreased vision. The most common problem is a need to change your glasses. Less common causes for vision changes are dry eyes, diabetes, cataracts, glaucoma, and macular degeneration. Many cases of blurred vision can be remedied by treatments other than MCS. It may be that you have suffered from eye strain, or are in need of a stronger prescription. In these cases, your eye doctor will be able to discuss his findings with you along with your treatment options. Remember, if you do indeed have macular degeneration, do not accept his poor prognosis.

Why doesn't my eye doctor know about MCS?

All eye doctors in practice today were told that macular degeneration is a progressive, mostly untreatable, and, certainly, incurable condition. Treatment approaches have focused primarily on wet macular degeneration, a condition caused by fluid leaking into the macula. These techniques have included laser surgery and more recently photodynamic laser therapy.

Microcurrent stimulation is a relatively new procedure for the treatment of the eye. Currently, only five medical doctors, including myself, have been involved with a preliminary study using MCS in the treatment of macular degeneration. Although the results of MCS in the treatment of wound healing and the treatment of pain have been published in many other types of journals, most eye doctors do not have the time to read much outside of their field. Although these studies have been available to the medical community, doctors are very slow to incorporate new information unless it involves surgery or drugs. Most eye doctors rely on formal, large-scale scientific studies and the publication of results in journals. Unfortunately these studies take many years to conduct and require even more time to be published. Large studies are expensive to conduct and analyze, and these expenses are often underwritten by drug companies. For Microcurrent Stimulation there is no such benefactor. This does not in the least diminish its effectiveness, however.

Where patients have been treated with Microcurrent Stimulation, all the testing centers have reported positive results, such as 60 to 80 percent of treated patients experiencing an improvement of vision. Dr. Rossen's FDA study is merely underway and it is hopeful that the preliminary results of these trials will be released by the end of this year. I hope that this book, Microcurrent Stimulation: Miracle Eye Cure and my first book, Healing the Eye the Natural Way: Alternative Medicine and Macular Degeneration, will educate eye doctors to recommend this treatment to individuals suffering from macular degeneration. Because there is no harmful aspect, and no viable alternative to this treatment, I cannot think of a good reason to withhold this option until large scale tests are completed.

What Conditions Respond to MCS?

In clinical practice, MCS has been shown to work very well in both the dry and wet types of macular degeneration. There seems to be a better effect in the treatment of the dry type, but, if you have the wet type, do not be discouraged. MCS will work, but it may take a little longer for you to achieve a change in your vision. I, as well as other investigators, have observed that MCS works very well in hereditary conditions of macular degeneration. Some of the most dramatic changes have occurred in young patients with Juvenile Macular Degeneration or Stargardt's Disease. Please read the exciting stories of patients with visual improvement in Chapter Four. Improvement has also been observed in patients with Retintitis Pigmentosa. There have also been reports of patients with retinal hemorrhage and retinal stroke responding to MCS. (Side effects include: local redness and irritation, light sensitivity and some mild discomfort after the treatment. These side effects last a short period of time. To date no long term side effects have been observed) Because of the low incidence and minor nature of the side effects and the demonstrated safety of MCS, I would recommend a trial treatment of MCS in any ocular condition which involves the retinal or has vascular involvement. You have nothing to lose!

MCS And Various Eye Conditions

Patients with earlier macular changes have the best prognosis with MCS. It is best to begin treatment while the retinal cells are dysfunctional, but retain their structural integrity. This state is when the visual cells still have their cellular structure but are unable to meet the daily demands of vision. MCS can rejuvenate and heal those cells which are not functional due to poor blood and energy circulation and patients will often experience a dramatic improvement in their vision. In more advanced stages of macular degeneration, the cells lose more and more their ability to function and begin to die. This causes the loss of retinal tissue and development of scar tissue. MCS has less effect at this stage of disease, but visual improvement does occur over months of treatment. There is some evidence that retinal tissue might be regenerated using MCS, however is still unproven.

The general rule that I use in making a prognosis is the starting level of vision. If the vision is 20/400 or better, and you are able to see the "big E" on the eye chart, the prognosis for visual improvement is very good. Seventy percent of patients in this group will have an improvement of their vision. Patients with vision less than 20/400 will have a less favorable response to the MCS treatment. This does not mean that MCS will not work. It means the treatments must be done for a longer period of time before visual improvement occurs. There are many other factors that affect the outcome. This is why it is important to be under the care of someone who is experienced in working with MCS.

The MCS Treatment Protocol

While it is quite easy to use the MCS unit, it is advisable to learn to use under the direction of a skilled practitioner. I ask each of my patients to have six to eight treatments in my office over a time period of four days. The patient's response to these twice-daily treatments is carefully monitored. The patient also becomes familiar with the treatment procedure in order to confidently undertake home treatments.

Most people quickly become acquainted with the home unit and feel comfortable with the treatments. If you have a disability, such as a tremor, you may need assistance from a family member or friend with your treatments. However, most patients are able to use the home unit without any difficulty. The new stimulator glasses which I have been making in my office also help make the treatment easier to self-administer.

It is best to treat your eyes with the MCS unit twice a day for the first three months. After this you can decrease the number of treatments to several times a week to maintain your level of visual improvement. When you begin using MCS, please consult with your eye doctor for the latest treatment protocol. I will also provide the latest protocol on my website at www.homeopathiceye.com.

While you are undergoing home treatment, I recommend that you have a eye examination every three months. It is important to monitor the changes in your retina and vision. It may be necessary during this time to adjust the frequency and the duration of your treatments. Most patients after 3 months can reduce the number of treatments to 3 to 4 per week. This will depend on the level of your vision and health of your retina.

Other therapies can help increase the success of MCS treatment. Excellent nutrition, as well as supplementation with appropriate nutrients, is essential. I have covered this topic very thoroughly in the book "Healing the Eye the Natural Way: Alternative Medicine and Macular Degeneration". Not only did I make dietary recommendations, I also gave specific advice about vitamins, minerals, herbs, and other supplements. Chapter 10 of this book covers two other highly effective methods for improving your vision. Chelation therapy and Homeopathic treatment can be used alongside MCS without any difficulty. Read these chapters to see whether you feel either one of these, or both, would help you in a synergistic way. Why not give yourself the best possible chance of recovering your vision and the freedom and pleasure it brings you?

Can MCS Help You?

| 7 | **Getting Acquainted with your Unit** |

In this chapter you will learn how to set up and use your Microcurrent Stimulation unit. All of the patients I have worked with have found the unit easy to use and the procedure very pleasant. I know that you will also feel this way about it. If you are a person who is somewhat apprehensive of equipment and devices, you may have to exert some will power to approach the unit and get it set up. Perhaps you might consider asking a friend or family member to go through the set up and stay with you for your first treatment. After that, I promise, you will feel like a pro. So, don't hesitate. Remember that you have in your possession one of the most effective ways to restore your sight and reverse your condition. When you think of it in this way, there is no reason to wait a minute longer.

The recommended protocol is to receive the first 6 to eight treatments in the office. These will be administered the same way that a patient self-administers after he/she is permitted to go home with the device. The investigator's responsibility will be to assure that the patients are competent with the device before releasing them to treat at home.

Treating Retinal Disease with MicroStim® 100

Setting up the device.

When you open the case containing your Microcurrent Stimulation unit, you will find several components. These are 1.)The MicroStim® 100 Stimulator 2.) The probe 3.) The connector wire 4.) The battery and battery compartment 5.) The sticky electrodes 6.) Blue box, paper shaft Q-tips brand cotton swabs

Take a few minutes to look at and examine rach of the components from your kit and the following illustrations.

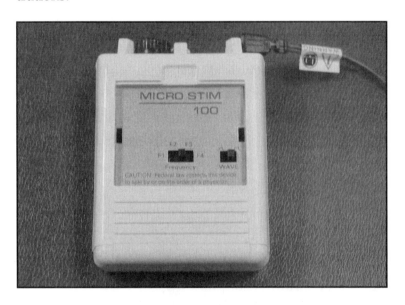

1.) The MicroStim® 100 Stimulator

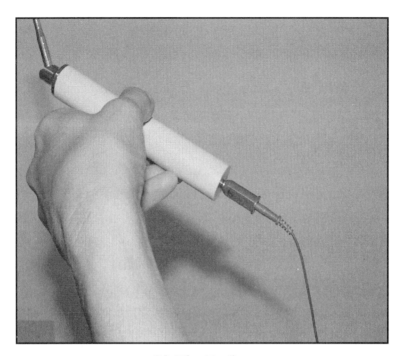

2.) The Probe

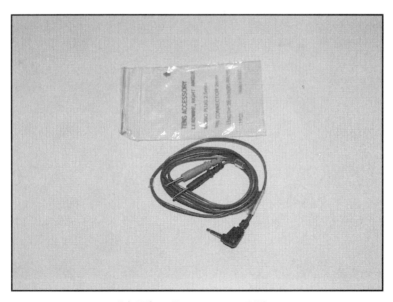

3.) The Connector Wire

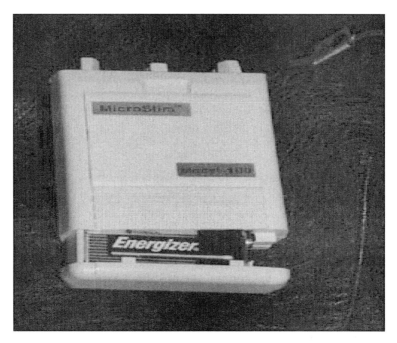

4.) Battery and Battery Compartment

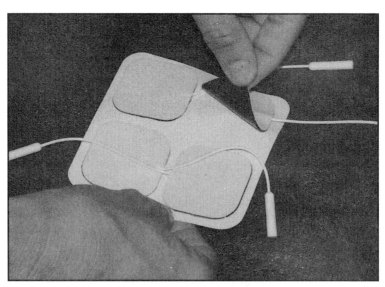

5.) The Sticky Electrodes

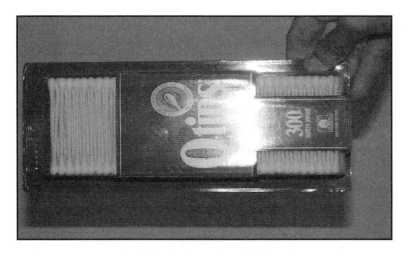

6.) The Q-Tips

Now, you will take the first two steps required for getting your unit ready for use.

> 1.) Take the stimulator and put in the
> battery. The alkaline battery enclosed with
> your unit is the only type of battery that
> you should use. Make a note to buy a bat-
> tery just like this one on your next shop-
> ping trip so that you have a spare. Insert
> the battery into the unit paying attention to
> the + and – terminals. Note that the bat-
> tery has a red colored + and – mark and
> diagram to help align the battery.

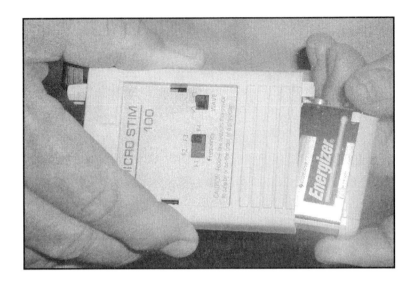

2.)   Plug the connector wire into the top of the MicroStim® 100. There are two holes on the unit.   Plug in the connector wire into the top of the unit.   You will find that the plug would only fit snuggly into only one of the holes, which is the correct connector hole. If you plug in the wrong hole, it will be loose and can easily come out.

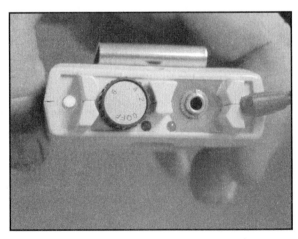

GOOD WORK!

Now we prepare to take the next two steps of set-up

3.) Select one of the sticky electrodes and plug the black pin of the connector wire into the white receptacle of the electrode wire and stick the ground electrode on the back of your hand on the same side as the eye you are treating. This completes the circuit with your eyes. This is needed to complete an electrical circuit on your eye. Remember that a ground is always necessary for treatment. A less expensive way to treat is to use a reuseable carbon electrode and a disposable electrode patch.

*Some units may have a Gold metal cylinder instead of the electrodes If you have the gold cylinder, plug the black pin into the connector on the cylinder.

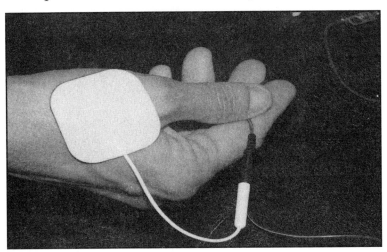

Getting Acquainted with Your Unit

The pads are applied to the electrode and the TENS wire is attached to the electrode like this.

Take one of the patches and remove it from the plastic backing.

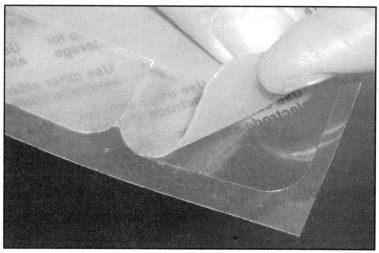

Plug the black pin of the TENS wire into the receptacle of the carbon pad.

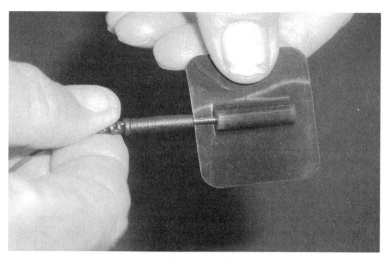

Attach the patch to the flat surface of the carbon pad and stick it to the back of the hand.

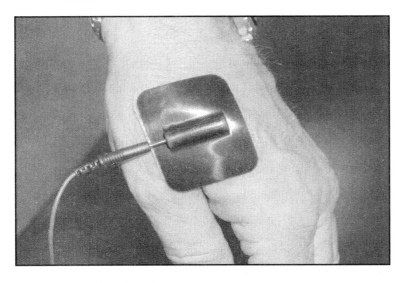

Connecting the Probe

4.) Plug the red pin of the connector wire into the red adapter on the bottom of the probe.

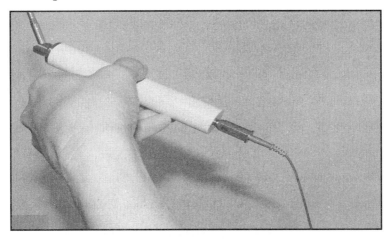

GREAT WORK!!

Now I will tell you how to use the Q-Tips to prepare for your treatment. You will get best results with Q-Tip brand cotton swabs. Use only the kind with the paper stems. Do not use plastic or wooden stems.

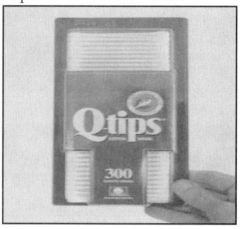

5.)   Set up the Q-tip.

Pick a Q-Tip from the box of Q-Tips. Break off the Q-Tip about 1/2 inch long and wet the head of the broken piece with tap water.

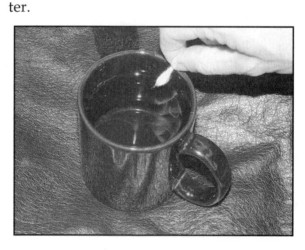

Insert the wet Q-Tip firmly into the end
of the probe using a twisting motion to
make it hold firm.

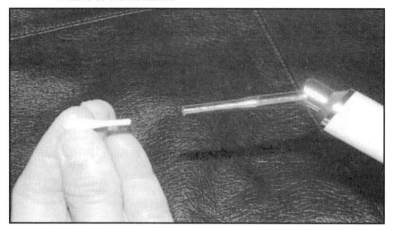

You are now ready to begin treatment. Feel free to drink
a large glass of water or juice before beginning in order to
relax.

The Treatment

Remove the door from the front of the MicroStim®
100 to reveal the controls. These are very simple to use,
and you cannot hurt yourself if you accidentally set them
incorrectly. Set the device frequency to F4 and then set
the Wave to SQUARE. Both switches are now set all the
way to the right. Remember Right is Right.

The eye treatment protocol is quite simple...

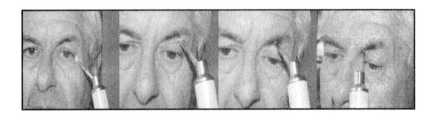

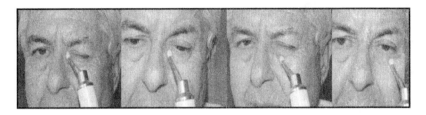

There are 8 points to treat on each eye as seen in the following diagram. Each point is to be treated 3 times per session. It does not matter with which point you start. In the following the diagram are 8 photos, showing each of the points being treated.   You will keep the waveform switch to the right at all times.   The frequencies you use will be F4, F3, F2, then F1.

Treating the 8 points.

You will keep the waveform switch to the right for all four steps. The frequencies you will use are F4 (292 Hz.), F3 (30 Hz.), F2 (9.1 Hz.), then F1 (.3 Hz.).

SETTING THE CURRENT IS CRITICAL: The current is adjusted by turning the knob on the top. (See picture of top control panel on page 110.) All the way to the left is off. Turn the knob clockwise until it clicks and turns on the device. Turning the knob clockwise from the numbers 0 through 6 increases the current.

With the current set all the way down to 0 (zero) touch the wet Q-Tip to one of the points around your eye. Then slowly turn the current up until you can feel it. Then turn it down until all sensation of electricity subsides. This is the setting you will use during treatment. Start each step with the current at 0 (zero). ALWAYS treat at a level where you do not feel any electrical stimulation. In this case, less is more.

Your treatment will consist of four rounds of point touching with the electrode. For each round you will set the frequency to a different setting. Each time you begin, se t the current down to zero and then slowly turn it up until you feel it. Then turn it down until you don't feel it for the treatment.

(1)   At the frequency F4 (292 Hz.), treat all 8 points on each eye for 15 to 20 seconds per point.

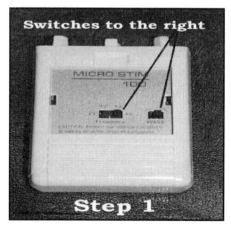

(2)   Set the frequency to F3 and the current down to zero. Then again slowly turn the current up until you feel it, then down until you do not feel it. Treat all 8 points on each eye for 15 to 20 seconds each.

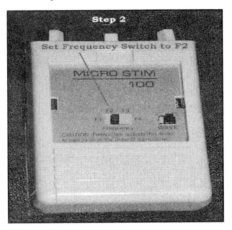

(3)   Set the frequency to F2 and the current to zero (0). Repeat the same steps as above. Treat all 8 points on each eye for 12 to 15 seconds each.

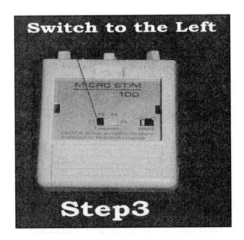

(4)   Set the frequency to F1 and the current to zero (0). Repeat the same steps as above. Treat all 8 points on each eye for 12 to 15 seconds each.

When you touch the points with the Q-tip, you will be touching inside the bone (orbit) on the closed eyelid such that, if the eye had been open, you would have been contacting the globe.

When you are treating, it is normal for you to experience what appears to be a flashing or a strobing effect. This is the effect of the stimulation of the retina and, although it may seem like there are lights flashing in the room, it is entirely internal and no one else can see it. The perfect setting for the current is where you can see the flashing but you can not feel the electricity. Not everyone sees the flashing.

In particular, many people either see no flashing or only see it at 9.1 Hz. (F2). It is important to see the flashing because that means that the retina is being stimulated. The flashing is usually most pronounced at the F2 and F1 frequencies, although different patients may be more sensitive to different frequencies. Most patients do not see the flashing at F4 or F3. Also, many patients do not see the flashing until after several weeks or even several months of treatment.

The Frequency of Treatment

Repeat the protocol described above once or twice daily for 60 to 90 days. After that, at least two two to three times weekly is still acceptable. You will want to have your vision re-checked in three months.

APPARATUS:

On the top of the device there are three lights, two jacks, and one knob. When you are treating, the red and green lights on the top of the device should all be lit and/or flashing. If they are not, there is a problem –the current is not getting to your body.

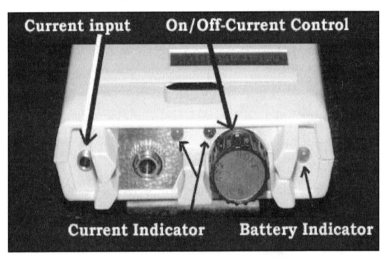

Current input   On/Off-Current Control

Current Indicator   Battery Indicator

Also important, the single green light on the top should be on and bright when the device is on. This light is the battery indicator. When this light starts to turn yellow or red, you must change the battery. A weak battery will not give an adequate treatment. Use only alkaline batteries. Rechargeable and heavy duty batteries are not acceptable. The power of these batteries is unpredictable and does not produce a consistent current with any batteries other than alkaline.

Notice: The MicroStim® 100 has an automatic 20-minute timer. This means that after being on for 20 minutes, the device will shut itself off. This will protect the battery from being drained if the device is accidentally left on after being used. When the unit stops after 20 minutes, if you wish to continue your treatment, turn the switch to off, wait about 10 seconds while the device resets, then turn it back on and your 20 minutes starts again.

NOTE: Please remember, the treatment of Macular Degeneration or anything other than pain is an off label indication for the MicroStim® devices and no claims are being made as to the efficacy of these devices for treatment of ARMD or anything other than pain. This protocol is to be used for experimental purposes only.

FDA Study of the effects of Microcurrent and Age Related Macular Degeneration

The study, to be done using MicroStim® 100i with glasses, is a prototype under FD investigation which we hope for approval by the end of the year 2000. These devises produce a unique micro-current waveform in the range of 10 microAmps through 3.5 milliAmps peak (True RMS AC + DC). The MS100i device is an automated version of the MicroStim® 400 (FDA 510 (k) number K890087C) stimulator that is FDA approved for the treatment of pain. It uses 2 MicroStim® LED Electrodes which are FDA approved for use with MicroStim® (FDA 510 (k) number 891107 A) electrical stimulators. The Led Electrodes are attached to the inside of a pair of glasses to deliver the stimulation to both eyes simultaneously. The glasses come in two varieties, one which has an electric band that connects the ear pieces to hld the glasses firmly in place and second which simply sits on the face and makes contact via gravity with the patient's head leaned back. The Eastern Electromedical IRB has evaluated this device. The opinion of the International Review Board is that the device is NSR (non-significant risk) and also MR (minimal risk). The treatment can also be done using a probe to traet specific points around the orbit. This probe is compatible with the Microstim® 100 and the Microstim® 100i. In this study, the treatment will be done using the glasses.

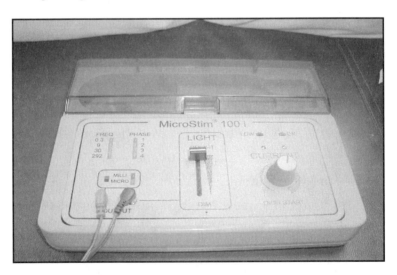

Front Panel of Microstim® 100i

Dr. Rossen has developed a new device for the treatment of carpal tunnel syndrome and macular degeneration. It has not yet been FDA approved and is not currently available to the public. At my request, he has been kind enough to provide me with the proposed treatment protocol and some pictures of the new device.

The following pages describe how a patient self treats with MicroStim® 100i. The first eight treatments in the office will be administered the same way that the patients will self-administer after they are permitted to go home with the device. The investigator's responsibility will be to assure that the patients are competent with the device before releasing them to treat at home.

(1.)   Set all controls to minimum See panel on page 112) and plug in the glasses to the appropriate outputs on the console.

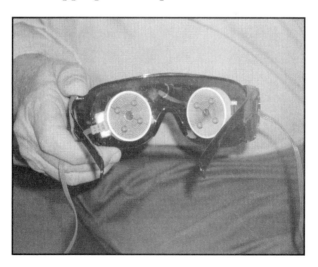

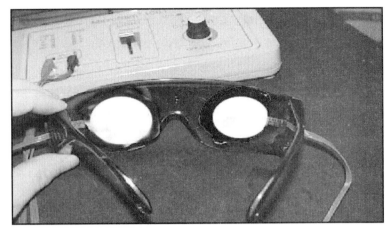

(2)   Wet the gauze sponges with sterile contact lens solution (or you may use tap water) and place the pads on the electrode surfaces, being sure that the two wet pads do not touch each other.

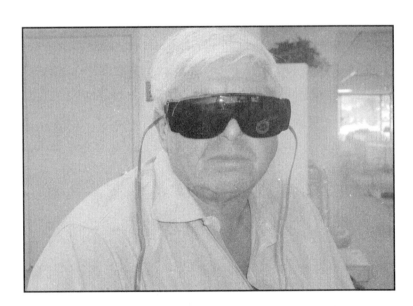

(3.)   Put on the glasses and lay back.

(4.) Start the treatment.

The treatment using the MicroStim® 100i is a four-step process. The steps 1.) 292 Hz., Biphasic square wave for one minute, 2.) 30 Hz., Biphasic Square wave for 1 minute, 3.) 9.1 Hz., Biphasic slope wave for 4 minutes and 4.) .3 Hz., Biphasic square wave for 4 minutes. No user intervention is needed for one step to the next, because the device changes its settings automatically. Once the treatment is started it will run for a total of ten minutes.

Time Out Mode

It is possible to take a break during the treatment for up to three minutes at a time. If you (the patient) need to stop, (say, to answer the phone, or something), just move the LED slider down to the bottom. The device will stop the timer cycle for up to three minutes and will begin again when you turn the light back on. While the MicroStim® 100I is in time out mode, the device will beep five times quickly every 15 seconds. If you leave the device in time out mode for more than three minutes, it will shut off and you will have to start treatment from step one. There is no harm to starting a treatment session over again.

Until the current is started, leave the light slide all the way down and turn on the device by increasing the current knob clockwise until it clicks and the on light comes on, and until you can feel the current and then turn it down until the sensation stops. Do not worry if you do not feel the stimulation. Some patients never feel it and sometimes you will feel the stimulation after you have completed a few treatments.

Next, increase the light slide until you can see the red light. Leave it set at a comfortable level. The treatment timer starts when you move the light slide up until the fast beep stops and the LEDs in the glasses illuminate.

When Step 1 begins, the device will beep one time. When Step 2 begins, the device will beep 2 times. When Step 3 begins, the device will beep 3 times and when Step 4 begins, the device will beep 4 times. When the treatment is complete, the device will beep 5 times and shut itself off.

That is the entire treatment.

Comparison of Microcurrent devices and TENS devices and other electrical stimulators.

As I have stated earlier in this book, the device I use is the MicroStim° 100, from MicroStim® Technology Incorporated in Tamarac Florida. The choice of this device was not a frivolous one. I have investigated the parameters which separate the valuable from the useless devices and I cannot more be stronger when I suggest that, should you decide to use microcurrent stimulation to treat your macular degeneration, stay with the MicroStim⁰ devices. It has been consistently effective in my practice and there has never been a single report of adverse response or injury. To my knowledge, every Ophthalmologist in the United States who is treating ARMD with microcurrent stimulation is using the MicroStim⁰ 100.

Most ophthalmologists will still tell you that there is no successful treatment for ARMD. There are dozens, if not hundreds, of electrical stimulators on the market. If just any electrical stimulator would work, surely everyone would know how to treat ARMD. One of the greatest dangers of using electrical stimulation for the treatment of macular degeneration could be the possibility of choosing the wrong device for doing the treatments. Electrical stimulators vary considerably from one to another, even when their specifications seem very much alike.

Dr. John Jarding, one of the first doctors to use microcurrent for treatment of ARMD, started by using the ElectroAcuscope, a $7000 microcurrent stimulator in his practice. In a scientific presentation to the International Association for Biologically Closed Electrical Circuits, Dr. Jarding reported that in 1995 his AcuScope broke down and the AcuScope Company told him it would take over a month to fix. They had no loaner device available for him to use, so Dr. Jarding called Dr. Rosen and borrowed a MicroStim⁰ 400 to use until his AcuScope was returned. Even though the AcuScope was then and is now one of the best microcurrent stimulators made for the management of pain, Dr. Jarding was so impressed with the response from the MicroStim®, that he immediately discontinued using the AcuScope in his practice and immediately began using only the MicroStim®. No matter how expensive or inexpensive, all microcurrent stimulators are not alike.

The MicroStim®100

The MicroStim is a patented, multi-frequency waveform generator that layers three simultaneous frequencies, one on top of another. Each frequency has a specific purpose which is critical to the safe and effective treatment of any physical problem, ARMD included. The MicroStim$^\circ$ 100 is designed to be as close to a perfect currents source as possible and that makes it not only different, but also superior for the treatment of ARMD.

The Current Source

Electricity and water flow in similar manners. While water and electricity do not have identical flow properties, the similarities can be used to create an understanding of the need for the specific type of current that the MicroStim provides.

While not mutually exclusive, there are two different types of electrical current flow devices. Devices are primarily categorized as being either of the current source or as being of the voltage source variety. The manner in which these two sources of electricity provide energy is very different. A device which provides a current source is more difficult to design and more expensive to produce.

To understand the difference between a current source and a Voltage source, let's take a look at how water flows, and create a garden metaphor for comparison.

There were two farmers who had each plowed an acre of land and sowed seeds of corn on their acres. Both were relying on the normally adequate summer rains to provide the essential water to their crops. The rains did not come, but both managed to arrange to pump water from the nearby river.

Each farmer's acre was very, very dry and the ground was hard. Both farmers knew that each acre needed four thousand gallons of water per day. The first farmer put a high pressure nozzle on his hose, and provided the four thousand gallons to his acre at high pressure in about 3 minutes. The second adjusted the nozzle to provide a fine mist for the whole day.

At the end of the day, the first farmer had completely ruined his field as the high pressure watering had disturbed all the soil and uprooted all the seedlings. The second farmer's field was perfectly watered by the fine mist that had gently saturated the soil without disturbing anything.

The difference between a voltage and a current source is similar to the difference between a fire hose and a soft Spring mist. A current source device, such as the MicroStim responds the changes in the electrical resistance of the body. Electrical resistance in the body is like the very dry soil which resisted the flow of water. A voltage source device would tend to blast through the tissue and disrupt nerve conductance, while a current source device tends to saturate the tissue with useful energy that the cells can use.

The old time TENS (Transcutaneous Electrical Nerve Stimulators) devices which were the first ones developed to manage pain, were simple voltage source devices. They were designed to block neurological transmission rather than the improve it. They made nerves work work work more poorly, not better. Properly designed microcurrent stimulators are designed to promote excellent transmission of neurological impulses by providing the energy which is missing in degenerated tissues.

Make no mistake, there are several types of devices that call themselves microcurrent stimulators. Some of these devices are built by companies who do not even know what microcurrent is. Some of the cheap units are nothing more than the old type of TENS voltage source devices which are designed to only work at the bottom 1 milliAmp of TENS range, more or less. These companies are simply trying to cash in on the remarkable effectiveness of a true microcurrent stimulator without even knowing what the technology is. You cannot tell the difference from the specifications. Only a series of specific complicated electronic tests will tell you if a particular device is a current or a voltage source device.

A properly designed microcurrent device cannot have a guarantee that it is putting out a specific current at a specific frequency because that is admitting that it does not change its' current and voltage in response to the changes in the patient's tissue resistance. For example, any device that states that it puts out 200 microAmps at a certain frequency must be avoided. It is simply not possible for a current source device to produce a stable current at any given frequency unless it has an unlimited Voltage range. Such a Voltage range would make that device quite dangerous and virtually impossible to run with a 9-Volt battery.

The Bipolar Pulse.

MicroStim provides a ½ Hz. biphasic or bipolar pulse that changes the direction of current flow once every second. This pulse is critical because uncontrolled direct current electricity can create electrode burns at the site that the electrodes contact the skin.

Electricity can cause burns by a process known as electrolysis. You may have heard of electrolysis because it is a process that is used to permanently remove unwanted hairs. During the process of electrolysis, a direct current runs down a hair and into the body, electrolytically burning and destroying the root or follicle of the hair. This destruction of the follicle is usually permanent and the hair does not grow back.

Up to a certain point, tissue electrolysis is reversible. MicroStim overcomes the tendency of the electricity to produce electrolytic burns by reversing the direction of current flow. The electrolysis that occurs each second is completely reversed in the following second. Although transient redness, lasting less than a hour, is often observed at the electrode site, there has never been a report of an electrode burn from MicroStim treatment using the patented biphasic pulse.

The Modulated Frequencies

As I mentioned, the MicroStim° has several different frequencies layered one on top of another. The first is the bipolar frequency, the second is the carrier wave. The 15,000 Hz. carrier wave is like the signals which you can use to tune a radio. It is a frequency that literally carries the other two frequencies into the body. A microcurrent device without a carrier of at least 10,000 Hertz cannot deliver the current deep into the tissues.

I feel the carrier wave is needed for the stimulation to go deep into the eyes and stimulate the optic nerve all the way into the brain. Remember that the optic nerve is part of the eye. Looking at it that way, the eye actually goes all the way into the brain to deliver its images.

Finally, there are the modulated frequencies. The MicroStim° provides four modulated frequencies. They are 292, 30, 9.1 and .3 Hz. There are actually two different types of modulated frequencies, those that produce electrical relaxation of the tissues and those that electrically energize or charge the cells. The 292 and 30 Hz. frequencies are the ones which relax or sedate the tissues and the 9.1 and .3 are the ones which energize or charge the cells.

As you know, I practice alternative ophthalmology. Many of the concepts of alternative medicine come from the Chinese medical arts or acupuncture and TCM or Traditional Chinese Medicine. In Chinese Medicine, there are two primary energetic states of tissue, congestion and deficiency. If these concepts seem foreign to you, in Western medicine we call them inflammation and degeneration.

The Chinese believe that energy travels in special pathways in the body and throughout the entire body. When the flow of this energy, which they call Chi and we call electricity, is in balance, the body works perfectly.

Certain conditions cause specific body tissues to develop high conductivity (high attraction to electricity) and to attract the body's electrical energy and make it pool and accumulate in massive quantities. When this happens, the body's tissues heat up and turn red. This common phenomena is known to us as inflammation. The Chinese physicians call it congestion. When tissue becomes congested, it prevents the flow of electricity to the surrounding or deeper tissues. This is in no way different from the process by which the element of a light bulb or a toaster releases heat and red light when supplied with ample electrical energy.

The MicroStim^{ö}'s two higher frequencies send pulses very rapidly in to the tissues to disperse the congestion. The tissues receive energy faster than they can process it and they fill up quickly with electricity. When they are filled up beyond their capacity to hold the energy, the suddenly discharge or release the excess energy. This phenomena is known as capacitive discharge. When this happens, the deeper tissues, the degenerative tissues, can receive their much needed energy because it is not all being wasted as it is turned to heat and light by the congested tissues. .

The lower frequencies. .3 and 9.1 Hz., are the ones which energize the tissues. They are like a biological trickle charger. The energy enters much more slowly and does not trigger a cellular capacitive discharge. Degenerated cells are like rechargeable batteries. They need to be periodically charged or they eventually die. The secret is to treat with the MicroStim$^{\circ}$ before they die, recharge the cells, and get them working again.

Finally – Considering Standard TENS

The FDA has always prohibited the use of TENS through the head. Standard TENS devices The idea of putting an old time standard TENS device on your eyes is simply a bad one. Do not do it. Microcurrent increases your cell's abilities to heal and produce protein. Standard or Millicurrent TENS actually does the opposite. It has been demonstrated to deplete the cell's ATP stores and slow down healing. This is exactly the opposite of what you want in a healing device. Just do not do it.

The Whole Microcurrent Enchilada

As you can see, as a microcurrent device, the MicroStim^Ó is a very complex and complete stimulator. Every aspect of its' design leads ultimately to a complete treatment. Leave any aspect out, and you only have a partial treatment which, at best, may provide some positive effect, at worst could cause problems which we have never experienced using the MicroStim® devices.

Getting Acquainted with Your Unit

8 Additional Points to Enhance the ARMD Treatment

By Damon P. Miller II, M.D., N.D.

In its most basic form the use of microcurrent stimulation for the treatment of retinal disease and other eye conditions is a local treatment, with the stimulating current applied only to points around the eyes. The use of the glasses with electrodes applies the stimulation only to the eye through the closed eyelids. In the protocol that I use for the treatment of macular degeneration and other degenerative retinal diseases, I instruct the people to stimulate specific additional points away from the eyes, for I have found that this adds to the effectiveness of the treatment. In this chapter, I will describe how these additional points on the arms, legs, body and ear are used and the rationale for their use. There will also be some discussion of how acupuncture can be used as a complementary procedure to enhance overall health and therefore the health of the eyes. An appendix at the end of this chapter will discuss the acupuncture theory behind the choice of the eye points that are the core of the treatment.

Additional Points to Enhance Treatment

Let me anticipate your question, "How can the stimulation of points on the arm or the leg or the ear affect my eye disease, or other problems I might have?" The desire of the Western scientific mind to want an answer to the question, "Why?" is very strong, yet there is so far a very poor understanding of why acupuncture works. The Office of Alternative Medicine at the National Institutes of Health has been studying acupuncture since 1995. In their first consensus paper on acupuncture in 1997, they concluded that the empirical data showed clearly that acupuncture works, but that the answer as to why it works would have to wait. To quote the National Institutes of Health, "While it is often thought that there is substantial research evidence to support conventional medical practices; this is frequently not the case. This does not mean that these treatments are ineffective. The data in support of acupuncture are as strong as those for many accepted Western medical therapies. One of the advantages of acupuncture is that the incidence of adverse effects is substantially lower than that of many drugs or other accepted medical procedures used for the same conditions."([1]) To quote one of my old acupuncture professors, " Don't bother asking why! Just use it (acupuncture) and if it doesn't work for you, don't use it anymore." I use it, and it works.

In the theories and understanding of health and disease upon which acupuncture is based, there is a very holistic view of a human being. The top of the body is connected to the bottom of the body, the inside is connected to the outside and the body and the mind and the spirit of a person are all a part of the same whole. The choice of points for an acupuncture treatment is a subject too complex to cover here, but typically, in addition to the treatment of local points around the eyes, the classical acupuncture treatment protocols call for the treatment of points away from the eye, on the body and on the arms and legs and hands and feet. As an example, one of the points included in many different protocols for the treatment of eye disease is a point called Bright and Clear which is point #37 on Meridian VII, the Foot Shao Yang meridian.

In Japanese acupuncture, there has been an extensive interest in the use of microcurrent stimulation as a form of Aneedleless acupuncture@, a stimulation therapy applied to the acupuncture points to treat a wide variety of diseases. There are two techniques from the Japanese that I use extensively, called Akabane testing and Ryodoraku therapy. Both of these techniques begin by first measuring electrical conductivity at specific acupuncture points. A sensitive instrument such as the MicroStim4007 is needed to make these sorts of measurements. If there are abnormalities detected, a treatment is given using either needles or a microcurrent stimulator to stimulate specific points. It is quite a remarkable thing to see how the simple insertion of an acupuncture needle or the application of a small amount of microcurrent stimulation at an acupuncture point on the forearm can change the electrical measurements at an acupuncture point on the foot. Following the treatment, which is pain-less, the measurements are repeated and the treatment is continued until the measurements are brought back to normal. There are many physicians in Japan who use these types of therapies as a sort of simplified acupunc-ture. I can testify from my own experience that these are quite effective therapies, though these procedures are more effective and powerful in the context of a more thor-ough and complete acupuncture treatment.

The MicroStim® 100 series of microcurrent stimu-lators for home use are not capable of making the mea-surements needed to perform the Akabane or Ryodoraku therapies. Still, from the extensive literature on these therapies it is clear that the stimulation of acupuncture points with microcurrent stimulation does produce an acupuncture-like effect. To enhance the therapy provided by the treatment of the points immediately around the eye, I instruct my patients to include in their treatment the stimulation of a series of points away from the eye. In addition, I stimulate a number of points on the ear, using theories taken from the French physician Dr. Paul Nogier. The French have refined the use of acupuncture points on the ear to a high degree and there are in fact acupuncturists who treat using ear points almost exclu-sively, with good results.

Selection of Points for Placement of the Ground Electrode

The use of microcurrent stimulation for the treatment of eye disease is not an acupuncture treatment, yet the development of the protocols for the treatment of eye disease relied in part on acupuncture theory. Acupuncture alone can be considered simply a form of stimulation therapy, and there have been extensive efforts to develop protocols of treatment using acupuncture needles for the treatment of various eye diseases. Treatments using acupuncture needles were actually mildly effective in the treatment of retinal disease but frequent treatments were needed which required frequent visits to a practitioner. With the significant advancements in the technology of the microcurrent stimulators, the treatment with microcurrent stimulation therapy has proven far more effective than the techniques with needles and has replaced them.

The microcurrent stimulation unit designed by MicroStim® Technology, Inc, is the unit of choice for all of the physicians I know that are treating retinal disease. The same specifications that make this unit so effective for the treatment of retinal disease make it an acceptable unit for use in the Japanese Aneedleless acupuncture@ techniques mentioned above. There are many inexpensive electrical stimulators on the market, and it must be emphasized that the majority of these are not adequate for the treatment of retinal disease or for use in the specific types of electrical acupuncture treatments I refer to above. There have been tremendous advances in the technology of electrical stimulation, and I cannot emphasize enough how important it is that you use the best technology possible if you wish to get the best possible results. An inexpensive machine could at worst actually do harm to your vision, and at the very least would provide ineffective therapy.

The current from all of the MicroStim® units is delivered as an alternating phase current, meaning that the polarity of the current switches each second. It is not important that you understand this, but the result of this design feature is that treatment is delivered at both the handheld probe on the MicroStim1007 and at the ground electrode. Since you are delivering treatment to the point where you place the ground electrode, there are particular ground points that I instruct people to use as one of the ways of providing some treatment at points away from the eyes. There are multiple points that I instruct people to use for the ground electrode and I advise them to choose a different point each day, as there are some mild but undesirable consequences of using the same ground point day after day. There is nothing unsafe about using the same ground point day after day, but over time, it can make the treatments less effective.

The seven points recommended for the place-ment of the ground electrode are:

1. Tao dao (Kiln Path), Point 13 on the Governor Vessel Meridian, located between the first and second thoracic vertebrae on the posterior midline. *(Figure 1)*

Figure 1

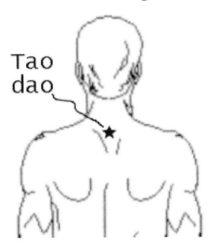

2. Wai guan (Outer Frontier Gate), Point 5 on the Arm Shao Yang Meridian, located two fingers' width above the wrist joint on the posterior forearm, between the radius and ulna, approximately where your watch would sit. (The point is found on both arms.) *(Figure 2)*

Figure 2

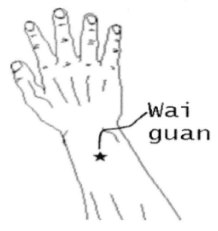

3.   Yin bao (Yin Envelope), Point 9 on the Leg Jue Yin Meridian, located one hand's width above the knee crease, on the medial surface of the thigh. (The point is found on both legs.) *(Figure 3)*

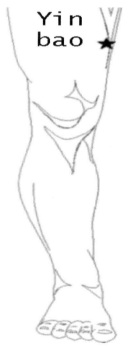

Figure 3

4.   Guang ming (Bright and Clear), Point 37 on the
       Leg Shao Yang Meridian, located about five inches
       above the ankle bone on the outer surface of the
       calf, at about the point where the top of your socks
       would hit. (The point is found on both legs.)
       (Figure 4)

Figure 4

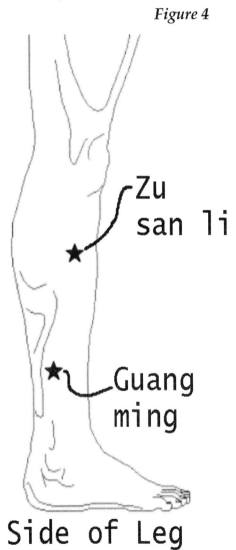

Zu
san li

Guang
ming

Side of Leg

Additional Points to Enhance Treatment

The following points are also possible points that could be used for placement of the ground electrode:

5.   Qi men (Gate of Hope), Point 14 on the Leg Jue Yin Meridian, located at the top of the abdomen on the inferior edge of the rib cage, in line with the nipple on either side. *(Figure 5)*

Figure 5

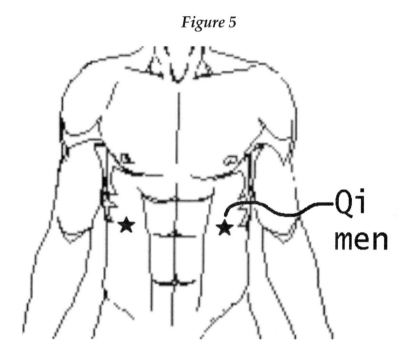

6.   Gan shu (Liver Correspondence), point 18 on the Leg Tai Yang Meridian, located two fingers width lateral to the midline of the back, at the level of the interspace between the spinous processes of the ninth and tenth thoracic vertebrae, on either side. *(Figure 6)*

Figure 6

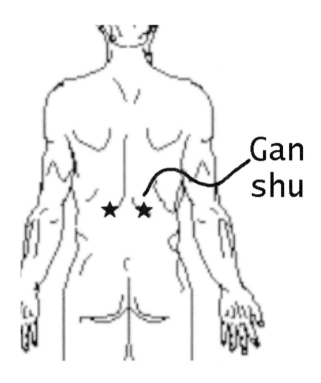

Points Away From the Eye to Include in the Treatment

What follows are points away from the eye that I include in the treatment. Treatment with microcurrent stimulation produces what the scientists refer to as a "field effect". This means that there are changes in the electrical properties of the entire body, no matter where the stimulation is applied. Electrical resistance in the tissues is lowered, and this is a beneficial effect. When you treat the points around the eyes, you can measure changes in the electrical resistance of the tissues of the feet. These electrical changes in the body are beneficial, but treatment of the eyes alone does not produce enough of this effect. For this reason, points are included on the neck and arms, which serve to enhance this effect for the entire body, which in turn has further benefit for the eyes. In addition, the treatment of the points on the back of the neck results in a decrease in the excess muscle tension that most people have in this area, which improves blood flow to the brain and eyes.

The addition of these points to your treatment may seem daunting at first, but don't despair. There are a finite number of points, and they are done in a very repetitive fashion so you will learn them quickly. You may want to consult with Dr. Miller or Dr. Kondrot or one of the other practitioners doing these treatments for help with learning the point locations if you have trouble with the instructions given here. I use these points with my patients, and I feel it adds to the success I have had in bringing improvement in vision using microcurrent stimulation for the treatment of macular degeneration and other retinal diseases.

Points on the Arm:

There are ten points in all, five on each arm. *(Figure 7).* There are three points at each wrist. One is in the center of the fleshy pad on the palm at the base of the thumb. The other two are on the wrist crease as shown on the diagram. There are two points on the inside of the elbow, at either end of the elbow crease. (See the diagram.) These points are named:

(1)   Yu ji (Fish Border), Point 10 on the Arm Yang Ming Meridian, located in the middle of the fleshy pad on the palm at the base of the thumb.

(2)   Da ling (Great Mound), Point 7 on the Arm Jue Yin Meridian, located in the middle of the crease on the palmar side of the wrist, between the palmaris longus tendon and the flexor carpi radialis tendon.

(3)   Shen men (Spirit Gate), Point 7 on the Arm Shao Yin Meridian, located on the crease on the palmar side of the wrist, in the depression on the radial side of the flexor carpi ulnaris tendon.

(4)   Shao hai (Little Sea), Point 3 on the Arm Shao Yin Meridian, located at the medial end of the elbow crease (Locate with the arm flexed)

(5)   Chi ze (Outside Marsh), Point 5 on the Arm Yang Ming Meridian, located at the lateral end of the elbow crease (Locate with the arm flexed)

Figure 7

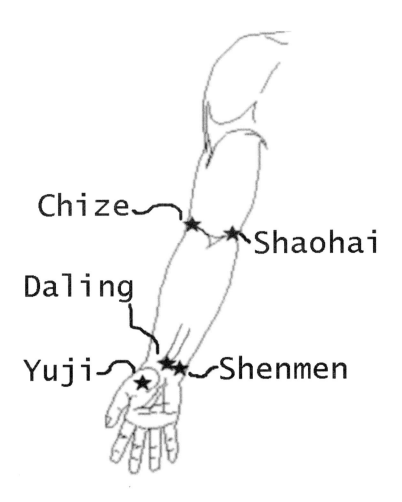

Chize

Shaohai

Daling

Yuji

Shenmen

Points on the Back of the Neck:

      There are ten points in all (five pairs), which are shown on the diagram. *(Figure 8)*. These points are named:

(6)   Tian zhu (Heavenly Pillar), Point 10 on the Leg Tai Yang Meridian, located one finger's width lateral to the midline on the back of the neck, at the

base of the occipital bone of the skull.

(7)   Feng chi (Wind Pond), Point 20 on the Leg Shao Yang Meridian, located lateral to Tian zhu at the base of the occipital bone of the skull, in the depression between the trapezius and sternocleidomastoid muscles.

(8)   Tian you (Heavenly Window), Point 16 on the Arm Shao Yang Meridian, located on the major crease across the rear of the neck, about two finger's width below the hair line, at a point three finger's width to the side of the midline of the back of the neck.

(9)   Bai lao (Hundred Labors), An Extra Point, located on the major crease across the rear of the neck, about two finger's width below the hair line, at a point one finger's width to the side of the midline of the back of the neck.

(10)   Ding Chuan (Calm Breath), An Extra Point, located one finger's width to the side of the midline of the back of the neck, at the level of the seventh cervical vertebrae.

Figure 8

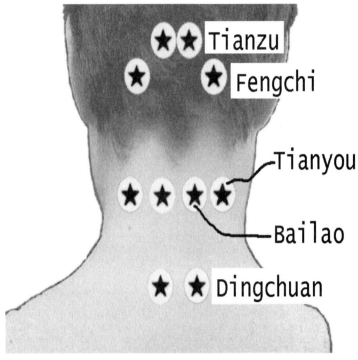

Back of Neck

An option for the treatment of the Back of the neck is to use the accessory probe with the mushroom shaped tip and some lubricating gel (such as Arnica Gel or Electrode gel). Gently massage the whole area on the back of the neck and the top of the shoulders. This can be very effective at relieving tension in this area, which can help to improve blood flow to the brain and eyes. Some people find this treatment of the back of the neck extremely relaxing, and choose to do it more often than once a week. It is fine and safe to treat these points away from the eyes more often if you choose.

Points on the Ear:

The ear points that I typically use are shown in the accompanying diagram. *(Figure 9)*. When I have the benefit of working with someone in my office, I often tailor these points to the individual but the 10 points shown would provide a good starting point for those who wish to include treatment of the ear points in their eye treatment protocol.

Only treat one ear at each weekly treatment. For example, if you treat the right ear one week, treat the left ear only the next week. (One option for choosing which ear to treat is to squeeze the earlobes. If one earlobe is more sensitive, treat the more sensitive ear.)

Figure 9

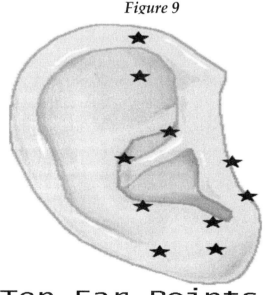

Ten Ear Points

Additional Points to Include in the Treatment:

There is a point on the midline of the face midway between the medial ends of the two eyebrows named Yin tang (Seal Hall) *(Figure 10)* which I include in the treatment of the eye points. After the eight points around one eye are done, this point is done. The eight points around the other eye are then done, followed again by this point. The eyes are treated three different times at three different frequencies, and as a result, this point gets treated for a total of six times during the treatment of the eye points.

Figure 10

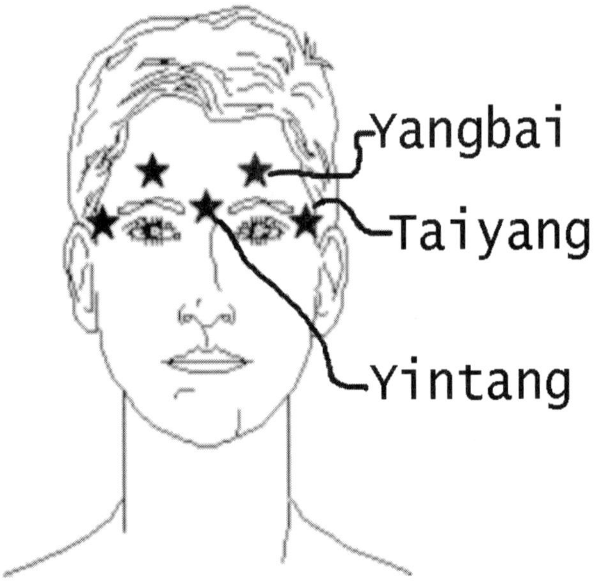

Yangbai

Taiyang

Yintang

When I am treating someone in my office, there are several points that I palpate, and if they are tender or sensitive, I instruct them to include these points in their treatment. Press firmly on the following points, and if you find any of them to be sensitive or tender, include them with the other points away from the eyes that you treat once a week. (See the diagrams that follow.)

(A) Yang bai (Yang White), Point 14 on the Leg Shao Yang Meridian, located on the forehead one finger's width above the midpoint of the eyebrow. (Figure 10)

(B) Tai yang (Highest Yang), An Extra Point, located in the middle of the temple, one finger's width behind and slightly below the lateral tip of the eyebrow. (Figure 10)

(C) Qi men (Gate of Hope), Point 14 on the Leg Jue Yin Meridian, located at the top of the abdomen on the inferior edge of the rib cage, in line with the nipple on either side. (One of the points for placement of the ground electrode) (Figure 5)

(D) Zu san li (Leg Three Miles), Point 36 on the Leg Yang Ming Meridian, located by placing ones palm over the kneecap. The point lies where the tip of the middle finger touches the lateral edge of the tibia. (Figure 4)

(E) Yong quan (Gushing Spring), Point 1 of the Leg Shao Yin Meridian, located on the sole of the foot in the crease that forms between the second and third metatarsal bones when the toes are flexed. (Figure 11)

139

Figure 11

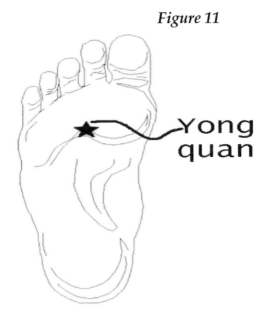

Yong quan

(F)   Xing jian (Walk Between), Point 2 on the Leg Jue Yin Meridian, located on the top of the foot in the space between the big toe and the second toe. (Figure 12)

(G)   Xia xi (Valiant Stream), Point 43 on the Leg Shao Yang Meridian, located on the top of the foot in the space between the fourth toe and the fifth (little) toe. (Figure 12)

(H)   Qiu xu (Wilderness Mound), Point 40 on the Leg Shao Yang Meridian, located in the hollow in front of the lateral malleolus of the ankle. (Figure 12)

Figure 12

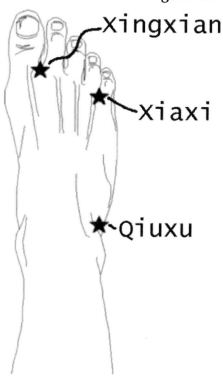

Classical Acupuncture as a Complementary Therapy with Microcurrent Stimulation

The care of your eyes and the repair of damage that comes as the result of years of degeneration require a body that is operating at its fullest and healthiest capacity. Microcurrent stimulation therapy is not a panacea or a miracle cure but a technology that can bring incredible improvements in the ability of cells of the eye to function and utilize energy and regenerate. As a result, the cells of your eyes work better, and you may see better. The body does not function as a set of independent organs and for this technique to be most effective, there must be an attention to a person's overall health as well as to the specific problems related to the eye. The many supplements that are used help to replenish and augment the many systems in the body that fight against oxidative damage and also provide the nutrients that are necessary for cells to repair themselves and maintain their structural integrity. Discussion of how a person can go further to maximize the overall state of their health in a way that will ultimately benefit their eyes is important if people are to derive the maximum benefit from the technology of microcurrent stimulation therapy.

Earlier, Dr. Kondrot has discussed the use of homeopathy in the treatment of patients he has seen with macular degeneration and other retinal diseases. Acupuncture and homeopathy are both systems of medicine which differ from Western allopathic medicine in how they view the cause of disease, as what they see as the underlying problem that needs to be addressed. Still, the reality is seen in the person with the disease. If you have a degenerative disease such as macular degeneration, that is the reality. You may talk about it with the language of homeopathy or with the language of acupuncture or consider it as Western medicine does with the language that speaks of an irreversible, progressive and untreatable disease. From the differing perspectives that acupuncture and homeopathy offer, come different ideas of how treatment might be approached and these differing approaches to treatments are often quite effective. Systems such as acupuncture and homeopathy consider disease in the context of the entire person and the treatments that derive from this perspective can be very useful.

When I include acupuncture as a complementary procedure to the therapy with microcurrent stimulation, I use either one of the simplified Japanese protocols such as Akabane Testing or Ryodoraku Therapy that I have described earlier, or a more thorough treatment with Classical Acupuncture

The system of Classical Acupuncture that I use when I treat people in my office is tailored to the needs of the individual that I am treating. I am constantly looking for what the person needs, and trying to provide that for them in the treatment. I do not treat everyone who comes to me for the treatment of their eye disease with microcurrent therapy with Classical Acupuncture, but if they live locally, and especially if they are troubled with various other medical problems, I strongly recommend an individualized course of treatment with acupuncture in addition to their treatment with microcurrent stimulation therapy. I do not feel that acupuncture alone is an adequate treatment for macular degeneration or other retinal diseases, for alone it does not bring the same successful results that I have had with microcurrent stimulation. For some people though, the addition of treatment with Classical Acupuncture has definitely brought further improvement in their vision.

Finally, there are many factors that affect health which are beyond the scope of this book but which are critical to a person's total health, mostly common sense, and which need to be at least mentioned. Exercise, a healthy and balanced diet and adequate sleep are critical to health. Maximum health is impossible if you are consumed by emotional or job related stress and it is prudent to learn techniques of stress reduction. If you have diabetes or other diseases that affect the vascular system, it is critical that these diseases be treated aggressively. Smoking tobacco in any form seriously compromises the small vessel circulation and anyone with retinal disease who smokes would be advised to stop. Alcohol is a toxin to the central nervous system, including the eyes and the use of alcohol should be done with extreme moderation. Studies that have shown some positive health benefits from an occasional glass of wine have demonstrated these benefits with as little as one glass of wine per week. Raw, unfiltered red or purple grape juice has been shown to provide similar benefits to wine. If you are still sexually active, a healthy sex life is important and you need to be open with your physician if there are problems with sexual dysfunction, since the most common cause of sexual dysfunction is the side effects produced by many prescription medications. In addition, many prescription drugs can have adverse effects on the eyes in someone with macular degeneration. Dosages can be adjusted and drugs substituted to minimize these unwanted effects, but only if your physician is aware that problems exist. In short, you need to have as your goal the best health possible.

APPENDIX:
Acupuncture Theory and the Points Used To Treat the Eye

Stimulation of the eight points around the eyes is the core of the treatment of retinal disease with microcurrent stimulation therapy. I include an extra point (Yin tang) described below. The points treated are all acupuncture points used to treat various eye diseases, and their names and locations are described below. There are excellent diagrams showing these points in the chapter describing the protocol using the Microstim 1007 unit with the hand held point probe.

The points are numbered, (Figure 13) and it is recommended that you treat the points in the order given. There are two reasons for this. First, the points Jing ming (Bright Eyes) and Tong zi lao (Orbit Bone) are two of the most useful points for the treatment of eye disease, and so it is desirable that they be done first. Second, it is good practice in doing a repetitive treatment like this to do the points in the same order each time. You will be doing this treatment daily, and it quickly becomes automatic. It is easy to let your attention wander, lose your concentration and forget where you are at in the treatment, and as a consequence, forget to do all of the points. For the sake of good habits, it is recommended that you always do the points in the same order, and the order given below is suggested.

The ninth point Yin tang (Seal Hall) is added because it provides especially strong and useful stimulation to the optic chiasm, the place where the optic nerves from both eyes come together behind the middle of the forehead.

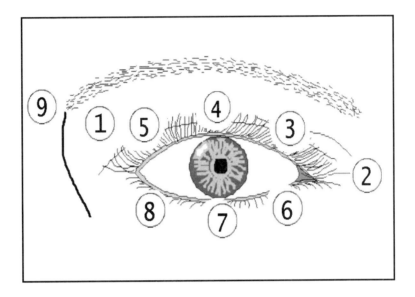

The treated points around the eye are named:

(1) Jing ming (Bright Eyes), Point 1 on the Leg Tai Yang Meridian, located in the hollow adjacent to the nose, on the upper lid just above the medial canthus of the eye.

(2) Tong zi liao (Orbit Bone), Point 1 on the Leg Shao Yang Meridian, located lateral to the lateral canthus of the eye on the rim of the orbit, which is the bony structure we refer to as the eye socket. All of the other points lie just inside the bony orbit, except Yang ming.

(3) Si zhu Kong (Silk Bamboo Hallow), Point 23 on the Arm Shao Yang Meridian, located on the upper eye lid midway between the lateral canthus and the middle of the upper eye lid, below the eye brow.

4) Yu yao (Middle Corner), An Extra Point, located at the midpoint of the upper eye lid, below the eyebrow.

(5) Zan zhu (Collect Bamboo), An Extra Point, located on the upper eyelid, midway between the medial canthus and the midpoint of the upper eyelid (Yu yao), just lateral to Jing ming (see above).

(6) Qiu hou (Behind the Hill), An Extra Point, located onand the middle of the lower eyelid, on the inner edge of the orbital bone.

(7) Cheng qi (Contain Tears), Point 1 on the Leg Yang Ming Meridian, located at the midpoint of the lower eyelid on the inner edge of the orbital bone.

(8) Dai jing (Surround Eyes), An Extra Point, located on the lower eye lid midway between the medial canthus and the midpoint of the lower eyelid (Cheng qi) on the inner edge of the orbital bone.

(9) Yin tang (Seal Hall), An Extra Point, located on the midline of the face midway between the medial ends of the two eyebrows.

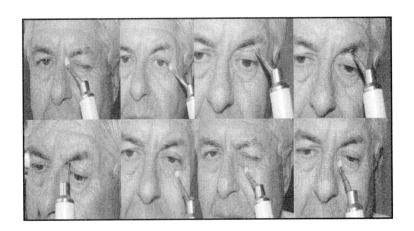

(Note that the trademark MicroStim® is used with the permission of MicroStim® Technology, Inc. The diagrams in this chapter and the material on the points away from the eyes is copyright ©1998, ©2000 All Rights Reserved by Damon P. Miller II, M.D., N.D., and is used with his permission.)

9

Other Uses of Microcurrent Stimulation

But can you dance to it?

What do dancing and MCS have in common? Herbert Berger would say: "Everything!" Herbie is a body worker as well as a doctor of Oriental Medicine. He has treated the injuries of the New York Jets, the Giants, the Knickerbockers, the 49ers, and, most recently, the New York City Ballet Company. Over the course of his twenty-one year career he estimates that he has treated, about 3000 patients. His clients have almost always been people who needed to recover as quickly as possible.

He uses MCS in the treatment protocol of 80 percent of his patients. "It is superb in the treatment of acute injury and muscle guarding pain," he states enthusiastically. In this chapter we will learn about the beginnings of MCS, the theory behind it, and the many types of injuries and chronic conditions that can respond to MCS treatment. Keep the names of these athletes in mind, since they have all benefited from Microcurrent Stimulation treatment for injuries that threatened to end their careers: Gary Carter, Mike Hayes, Joan Benoit, Joe Montana, Mike Spinks, and Mike Elkins

The Body Electric

Robert O. Becker published a book in 1987, titled The Body Electric. He was criticized by the medical profession for re-opening, in a major scholarly work, the subject of electrical energy, the body, and healing. Yet, prior to the early part of this century, healing through the use of electric therapy was quite well-accepted. As the world of medicine became more focused on proof and scientific explanations, biochemistry came to dominate as the most valid form of treatment. We must not overlook the fact that this coincided with the development of synthetic chemical products, including drugs. The economics of medicine will favor pharmacology over electricity for treatment. A patient with an electrical stimulator needs only purchase the correct batteries, plug it in, and use it as needed. A patient who requires drugs, on the other hand, may purchase the same medications over and over for the rest of his life. Drugs are a much more lucrative business for the medical industry.

Interestingly, although medicine by and large repudiates the idea of electrical forces in the body, chemical formulas are based on an understanding of atomic theory – that matter is composed of positively and negatively charged atomic particles. Chemical bonding is the result of atoms attempting to stabilize themselves by combining with other atoms. It makes sense, then, to postulate that all of life is composed of 'charged' matter. This includes the human body, all of its tissues, cells, and fluids.

When atoms combine with each other, they exchange electrons, the negatively charged outer elements in their shells. This flow of electrons from one atom to another is called current and it goes on continuously within the bodies of all living things. Some scientists believe that there are specialized cells that are responsible for conducting current. These cells move rapidly to the site of an injury in order to promote healing. Studies have measured an increase in both resistance and conductivity at injury and amputation sites. This tends to return to normal after healing is underway.

When researchers have attempted to manipulate the flow of electricity to injury sites, they have repeatedly discovered that a low current is most useful to enhance healing. In fact, research done in Europe has demonstrated that a relatively strong current can disrupt the healing process. That is why, in Microcurrent Stimulation, the flow of current is imperceptible to the person being treated, although it is strong enough to have a healing effect. Nevertheless, it is still difficult to understand how current works to promote healing. In fact, many physicians who used these devices were severely ridiculed by the medical establishment because they were unable to produce a theory to support their results. Remember, when we heal naturally, we do not feel the current moving in our bodies. This treatment is an attempt to simulate natural healing.

Cell Regeneration

All healing involves cell regeneration. Due to our ability to visualize biological processes through electron microscopes, we know a lot about how this happens. At the site of an injury, tissue usually develops a strong resistance to current, the natural current that circulates throughout the body. If there is inflammation, the inflamed tissue will be highly conductive and will attract the body's current in excess and redirect it so that it cannot move to the injured tissue. Wound or injury treatment requires that the inflamed tissue is healed enough to allow energy (electrons) to get to the deeper or electrically deficient tissues. If there is edema, the fluid in the tissue acts to block current flow and must be dispersed in the first step. Treatment with micro current is a way of doing what the body would do normally if it were perfectly healthy, and a way to do what the body is attempting to do in a faster way. It simply boosts the natural electronic process.

How to Treat Conditions with MCS

Once you have your MCS unit, you will undoubtedly find many ways to use it in addition to healing your vision. In Chapter 3 you read about how Grace Halloran used MCS to speed up and enhance the healing of her son's shattered elbow. This is an example of a way to use MCS for acute injuries. Acute conditions are those that arise suddenly and require immediate attention and care. They usually resolve completely. Chronic conditions also respond to MCS. Chronic conditions are those that are longstanding and/or recurrent. Examples are arthritis (longstanding) or tennis elbow that flares up after exercise (recurrent). Back pain and headaches are also examples of chronic conditions.

Herbie Berger, whose entire practice is devoted to helping injured athletes and performers to get back in the game or the production, described how he would treat a sprained ankle with MCS. His plan involves a first phase to reduce swelling and pain and then an ongoing set of treatments until the ankle is healed.

"First of all move the probe of the unit around the periphery of the injury to disperse fluid out of the edematous area. This can take from 20 to 40 minutes. Then move closer to the injured site and treat the acupuncture points in the area. Any point on the skin can be treated successfully, but we know that acupuncture points are on meridians that conduct the life force."

Following the first treatment, you will want to treat the area once or twice daily. You should be able to recognize that the injury is healing by reduced swelling and pain, and return to normal use. Treating a healing injury or a chronic condition usually requires daily use of the unit for a week. The number of treatment sessions can be one or two. Evaluate the results after a week to be sure that you are getting good results.

Chronic conditions also require daily treatment for at least a week. Conditions known to respond to MCS are occipital headache, chronically cold extremities, lower back pain, and hip and knee pain. Other conditions that may be helped are carpel tunnel syndrome, tennis elbow, burns (treat only around the area, not directly on the tissue) and adhesions. A condition such as a headache can respond to daily treatment of the affected area even if there is no headache present. The increased circulation and decreased muscle spasm in the neck produced by MCS will help reduce the intensity of, and perhaps prevent, future headaches.

The best way to treat an area, according to Herbie Berger, is to treat the area surrounding the painful part, rather than right on the affected joint or limb. He adds that soft tissue is more responsive than bone, so place your probes on well-padded areas. For example, if you have knee problem, treat the back of the knee and the surrounding tissue rather than directly on the kneecap.

The Future of Microcurrent Stimulation

The future that I am most interested in for this technique is the restoration of sight in individuals with macular disease. However, there are many other applications for this method, and exciting research is ongoing in many areas of medicine. The use of current to heal bone has become standard in orthopedic medicine. Doctors have come to accept the existence of electrical current in the brain and heart, and they routinely use electroencephalograms and electrocardiograms to study the brain and heart function respectively. In addition to wound healing and pain relief, one of the most exciting areas investigating microcurrent is in limb and organ regeneration. What if new cartilage could be grown in arthritic joints? What if a diseased organ could be replaced by a new one regenerated within the individual who needs it? We watch in amazement as salamanders grow new limbs when one is amputated. Scientists who have studied this phenomenon have discovered that there is a high degree of current conductivity at the site of salamander stumps, and they believe this is responsible for the regeneration. For the most part humans do not have limb regeneration capacity, although it is known that children under eleven years of age can regenerate fingertips that have been lost.

I firmly believe that the future of medicine is in electrical therapy, especially Microcurrent. We have just about reached the limit of the 'combat' approach where disease and disability are viewed as the enemy; drugs and surgery are the 'good guys', and the war is waged over and over again. This results in far too many casualties. It is time to work in concert with the energy and forces for healing that we have in our own bodies and use them to stay healthy and repair ourselves when illness and injury occur.

As the owner of a microcurrent unit, consider yourself a pioneer in self-care for the eyes and many other injuries and disabilities for yourself and your family members.

Other Uses of MCS

10 | Better Nutrition Improves Your Results

How Microcurrent Stimulation Works

In an earlier chapter I described, in some detail, the mechanics of Microcurrent Stimulation. I also talked about the way the electrical field of the body is involved in Microcurrent Stimulation. In this chapter, I will talk more specifically about the need to pay attention to the quality of nutrients in the body in order to deliver the highest quality material to the eye and surrounding tissue.

First, join me on a short tour of the interior of your body. We all know that we must eat to live, but few of us think about the way what we eat is delivered to all the cells in the body. When we ingest food, it is broken down into an easily assimilated liquid form. The unusable part of the food is eliminated through the bowels. The usable part is absorbed into the blood stream through the walls of the small intestine. From here it is delivered to the liver where further purification occurs and where specialized liver enzymes either break down or store excess fat and sugar molecules. A final purification takes place in the kidneys where waste material is filtered out of the blood and removed from the body via the urine. Other organs of detoxification include the breath and the skin. Perspiration is one of the ways that toxic material from the lymph system is eliminated.

Life-supporting nutrients are delivered to cells, organs, and tissues by the circulatory system. This is composed of veins, arteries, and capillaries. It is a transport system whose own physical and biochemical integrity is as important as the material it transports and the medium within which it is transported. Looking first of all at the system, we see the need for clear, unobstructed vessels, with elastic walls. It is well known that very few individuals past middle age have such a system. It has also been demonstrated, that health can be restored to the circulatory system through lifestyle changes. Within the transport system is the transport medium, or blood. The chemical composition of the blood is the result of its own make-up, namely the red and white blood cells as well as the material that is carried by the blood, such as iron, and the material that is dissolved in the blood in the form of nutrients. No amount of good nutrition can overcome the toxic load found in the bloodstream of people who cannot digest or assimilate properly or who have a sluggish liver or pancreas.

The second transport system in the body is the lymphatic system. This is composed of the lymph channels and the lymph nodes. It has two functions. The first is to remove excess fluid from the spaces between the cells and transport it to the veins for reuse or elimination. The second function is to screen and filter out harmful material like viruses, bacteria, and cancer cells. Lymph nodes provide a kind of way station for the action of the white blood cells and other 'attack' units produced by the blood. Unlike the circulatory system, which is propelled by the action of the heart's beating, the lymphatic system is passive. It is moved by the action of the muscles and surrounding tissue. This is why exercise and motion in general is so important to immune system functioning.

We can now explore how both of these transport systems work in Microcurrent Stimulation. The circulatory system carries nutrients to the tissues of the eyes as it does to all other parts of the body. When the low voltage of Microcurrent Stimulation is applied to the tissues around the eye several events occur. Investigators have shown that microcurrent improves cells' ability to utilize nutrients. Studies have shown that in addition to nutritional elements being moved into the cells more easily, there also appears to be an improvement in the circulation. The current travels through the skin to the underlying blood vessels. The blood flow is quickened or refreshed by the impulse and begins to move at a slightly faster pace, making nutrients more readily available to the surrounding tissue.

At the same time, the exchange of nutrients between the capillaries, or tiny outlets of the veins and arteries, is speeded up. This carries accumulated waste away from the areas of the cells of the eyes and deposits it in the nearest lymph channels for removal. Lymph nodes surround the eye socket, giving the appearance of a small chain. As the tip of the Microcurrent Stimulator touches these, they respond to the pressure as well as the electrical input and come alive.

All this activity is good and refreshing to eye tissue. However, the components of the fluid that are carried to the tissue are of great importance. Since we are stimulating the flow of material to eye tissue, the more nutrient-rich it is, the better. Depleted blood will not improve the health of the area. Toxic blood, loaded with unusable material, will result in a greater toxic load for the immune system to handle. All the patients I have treated successfully with Microcurrent Stimulation have improved their nutrition as part of the program. I consider this essential. In fact, I would venture to say that a person who is unwilling to improve their nutritional status would be better off not using Microcurrent Stimulation. The reason for this is that it could be harmful to stimulate the circulation to the eye if the quality of the fluids that will bathe the eye tissues is poor. In fact, it may result in speeding up of the very disease process you are hoping to arrest or reverse.

What is Good Nutrition?

There are several components of good nutrition. For a healthy person, a good diet and a program of supplements at maintenance level are enough. For a person with a chronic or degenerative disease, good nutrition is more complex. It certainly entails a good diet as a starting point. The program of supplementation needs to be at a higher level in order to act therapeutically against the disease process. A third component is an enhanced anti-oxidant program to counteract the effect of the so-called free radicals produced by cellular metabolism. In addition to vitamins and minerals, three herbs need to be included: Bilberry, Euphrasia and Gingko Biloba.

By following the recommendations given in this chapter, you will embark upon a total healing program that will assist you in healing your eye disease as well as any other degenerative and chronic diseases you may have.

Diet

In changing your eating habits, keep two maxims in mind. First, change slowly; second, think in terms of adding good food rather than 'taking away' your unhealthy favorites. A bit of explanation is in order regarding these suggestions. Changing slowly is apt to result in a more permanent commitment to a lifetime of good eating habits. I suggest trying one new vegetable and one new grain each week for several months until you find that you have significantly expanded your repertoire of foods. As you do this, you will discover the wisdom of the second maxim. By adding new foods and changing you body's chemistry, you will find that your old cravings begin to fade away. Some of the sugary or salty snacks you were accustomed to eat will begin to feel too sweet or too salty.

You will want more moderate tasting food. Alcohol, coffee, and other stimulants will begin to feel too overpowering to the milder, calmer state induced by simple, nutritious food. Eventually, of course, you will need to become aware of overindulgence in fat, sugar, salt, alcohol, and caffeine, and confront it directly. But, for the beginning phase of diet improvement, just focus on adding new, nutritious foods

Then the question is: "What to add?" A nutritionally sound diet is based on whole foods, that are as unadulterated as possible. This means increasing your consumption of produce and whole grains that are organically grown. Organically grown means grown without chemicals. Ingesting toxic chemicals places a huge burden on the detoxification processes of your organs and lymphatic system. You recall the description of how circulating fluids carry nutrients to the eye, and how these fluids are speeded up with Microcurrent Stimulation. If these fluids are contaminated with pesticides, herbicides, and preservatives, they are not going to help your vision very much.

You will probably need to alter your shopping habits. Organic produce can be found in health food stores and, often, at Farmers' Markets. Do some research about where these resources exist in your community and begin to patronize them. Health food stores are also the source for grains – the other staple of a healthful diet. Health food stores often have good quality meat, poultry, fish and eggs available as well as other forms of protein such as tofu and soy products. You can skip the packaged and processed foods here just as you will skip them in regular markets. Margarine and coffee have been found to be particularity toxic to the macular tissue, and I urge you to give them up completely. The world of natural, nontoxic foods is very complex and colorful. There are fine cookbooks on the market to help you make this transition. One emphasis that is essential for persons with macular degeneration is to add lots of leafy green vegetables, especially kale, collard greens, and spinach. While these may not be emphasized in the cookbooks, it is important that you make your own adjustments in menus to include them. I'll say more about these a bit further on in the chapter when we discuss Lutein and Zeaxanthin.

Digestion

It has been found that many people who develop degenerative eye disorders also have poor digestion. In some cases digestion may be so severely impeded that they have developed Crohn's disease or irritable bowel syndrome. Digestive enzymes produced by the liver and pancreas and hydrochloric acid produced by the stomach are diminished as we age. Feeling bloated, gaseous, or experiencing heartburn after eating are some of the signs of poor digestion. If you have these symptoms with any regularity, you need to support your digestion with enzyme supplements and hydrochloric acid. This will help the nutrients become bio-available for your body to use so they do not pass out as undigested waste. Many people, particularly the elderly and those with chronic illness, have "leaky gut" syndrome. This means that nutrients from food pass through without being absorbed in your bloodstream and circulated to the organs and tissues that need them so desperately. A deficiency of bile salts may also affect the body's ability to absorb fat-soluble vitamin A. Light-colored stools may be a sign of low levels of bile salts. Supplements should be taken if this condition exists.

A toxic condition results from the build-up of cellular waste in the body. This is one of the major contributing factors to the development of Macular Degeneration. Traditional means of detoxifying included enemas, saunas, fasting and the use of colonics to rid the body of waste through the normal channels of the colon and skin. Research into the dynamics of detoxification have resulted in the production of organ stimulating supplements, herbal cellular and bowel cleansing furmulas that are highly effective in ridding the body of wastes and setting the stage for optimal nutrition.

Supplements

Many people resist the idea of taking supplements because they believe they can get all their nutrients from their diet especially if you have a degenerative disease, such as macular degeneration, this is simply not true. Your body has already demonstrated its inability to maintain a healthy state on food alone. The fact that you have developed a disease is, in my opinion, the proof that you need higher quality and a greater quantity of nutrients.

The most important type of supplements you require are those called the anti-oxidants. These are the vitamins and minerals that counteract the damage to tissue electrons by free radicals that are released during metabolic processes. When these are allowed to circulate, they damage surrounding tissue. Anti-oxidants are 'free radical scavengers.' This means they seek out and destroy or neutralize free radicals. I will review the major anti-oxidant vitamins and minerals below, and then suggest a way that you can get most of your supplement needs met without taking a lot of pills.

Vitamins
Vitamin A

This was the first vitamin discovered; hence its name. It is also called retinol because of its importance in vision, especially in night vision. It is also very important in the formation and maintenance of healthy skin, internal tissues, bone, and hair. Pre-formed Vitamin A is available in cod liver oil and in the liver of animals as well as in dairy products. Vitamin A is fat soluble, and it is stored in the liver, kidneys, lungs, eyes, and fat tissue. It needs Vitamin E to expedite absorption and Zinc in order to release it for use in the body. Pro-vitamin A as beta-carotene is available from orange, yellow, and green vegetables and fruits. Because this nutrient is stored in the body, it is possible to develop Vitamin A toxicity characterized by dry skin, nausea, and loss of appetite. Pregnant women should not consume large doses of Vitamin A. Many people like to avoid the Vitamin A toxicity problem by taking Vitamin A as beta-carotene, a substance that converts to Vitamin A on an as-needed basis. This is a fine idea – as long as you have a normally functioning thyroid. Some researcher's think that a large number of people cannot convert beta-carotene to Vitamin A because they have hypothyroidism, an under active thyroid. Still other scientists think that a large percentage of people with macular degeneration have hypothyroidism, regardless of whether it has shown up on their blood tests or not. I have come to regard Vitamin A deficiency as contributory to macular degeneration. Therefore taking Vitamin A should be part of a complete nutritional program.

Beta Carotene

This nutrient, found abundantly in foods, is a Vitamin A precursor. This means that it converts readily to Vitamin A in the body as the body's requirement for Vitamin A demands it. It is water-soluble, unlike Vitamin A, which is stored in fat tissue. Specific foods contain types of beta-carotene known to support the health of the macula. When you add these to your diet regularly, you are adding a good source of beta-carotene from food.

Vitamin C

Vitamin C is perhaps the most accepted and well

known supplement. The federal government is in the process of revising the Recommended Daily Allowance upwards of the current 60 milligrams. As a balance to this, recent studies have shown that the large doses of Vitamin C recommended over the past years by some specialists in natural health may be unwarranted. Human beings are not able to create Vitamin C, as are most other animals. It is water soluble and you cannot store it to use later. It must be obtained on a daily basis from food and supplements.

Vitamin C's main function in the body is to strengthen collagen, the fibrous material in the skeleton and surrounding each cell. It also aids in the production of thyroid hormone and in lowering cholesterol. Because it strengthens the cell walls, it is an anti-oxidant par excellence since strong cell walls prevent damage from free radicals.

Vitamin C supplements come in many forms. When combined with calcium and magnesium and/or potassium, it can be soothing to the stomach rather than irritating. Ester C is a form of Vitamin C that is well tolerated by many people, even if they experience stomach distress with other forms of Vitamin C. If you experience diarrhea from taking vitamin C, reduce your dosage. Orange juice is a good source of Vitamin C. The orange juice with added calcium also seems to be less upsetting to the stomach.

Vitamin E

The food sources of Vitamin E are grains, seeds, and nuts. Wheat germ oil is an especially rich source. Vitamin E works to protect and enhance the cell membranes of the skin, eyes, and liver from free radical damage. It is a fat-soluble vitamin, like Vitamin A, and is absorbed from the intestines and stored in the liver and fatty tissue, heart, and muscles. It is not as stable in the body as Vitamin A, and more is lost through excretion. It was formerly believed that d-alpha tocopherol was the best form, but current thinking favors mixed tocopherols. Much less valuable is the synthetic form, dl-alpha tocopherol. I do not recommend this.

Minerals

Chromium

Although chromium is needed in minute quantity in the body, a deficiency may lead to serious metabolic disorders. Diabetics almost all show a deficiency of Chromium. It plays an important role in balancing blood sugar (glucose) levels and this contributes to the health of blood vessels. A chronic chromium deficiency is most likely due to depleted soil and over processed food. Fortunately most multiple vitamin and mineral supplements contain the amount needed on a daily basis.

Selenium

Selenium is another micronutrient. Its deficiency is also associated with depleted soils. The amount of selenium in the soil and water of an area can vary greatly. However, conservative levels of selenium supplementation is generally considered safe. The lens of the eyes of patients with cataracts have shown far lower levels of selenium than are required in healthy tissue. This suggests a strong association between eye health and selenium levels. Selenium needs Vitamin E to perform its antioxidant functions; I recommend that you take both of these nutrients.

Zinc

Zinc is another mineral diminished due to poor soil conditions. An added problem in obtaining adequate zinc is that meat and animal foods are the most abundant sources. We are recommending a diet high in produce and grains and lower in animal products. Yet virtually all the tissues in the body need Zinc. The retina contains the second highest concentration of zinc in the body (male sexual organs the highest.) Zinc is also necessary to transport Vitamin A to the eye, and to stimulate cellular metabolisms that will combat free radical damage.

As important as it is to obtain adequate amounts of zinc, by far the greater problem is how easily it is depleted through sweat and stress. Zinc is depleted in metabolizing many commonly prescribed drugs for hypertension, high cholesterol, and many other conditions. Anyone taking these drugs should be certain to supplement with zinc. Like Vitamin A, Zinc can also be toxic if the dose is too high.

Essential Fatty Acids
DHA

Both Omega-3 and -6 Fatty Acids are essential nutrients for normal development in mammals. Omega -6 Fatty Acids are necessary primarily for growth, reproduction and the maintenance of skin integrity. Omega -3 Fatty Acids are involved in the development and function of the retina and cerebral cortex and other organs such as the testes.

Docosahexanoic acid (DHA) and eicosapentaenoic acid (EPA) are essential Omega-3 Fatty Acids found in aboundance in cold water fish and their oils. DHA is an essential nutrient for achieving optimal brain and eye function. It comprises about 60% of the rod outer segments in the photoreceptor cells. Brain tissue is about 60% fat, 25% of which DHA. DHA levels correlate with visual and mental performance and several Neurological and visual disorders, including retinitis pigmentosa.

Cells in the retina, brain and other parts of the nervous system have connecting arms that transport electrical currents, sending visual information from the retina to the brain and messages from the brain throughout the body. DHA supplementation ensures the optimal composition of cell membranes necessary for the most effective transmission of these signals. Plentiful stores are needed and a daily dose of approximately 500 mg daily is recommended.

A 1990 study demonstrated that DHA with EPA given in the form of fish oil exerts a beneficial dose-dependent effect on coronary circulation with reduced trig-lycerides, total cholesterol, and blood pressure while causing no significant increase in bleeding. It's use in wet macular degeneration is unparalled since its main work in the body is to heal and support blood vessel walls.

Evening primrose, borage and black currant oil are good sources of Omega –6 essential fatty acids including gamma-linolenic acid (GLA). Supplementation with GLA may offer a method to bypass the disturbance in Omega –6 essential fatty acid metabolism associated with diabetes and diabetic retinopathy.

Taurine

And, finally, I need to mention Taurine. Taurine is a sulfur-containing amino acid, which is found naturally in egg whites, meat, fish and milk. High concentrations are found in the heart muscle, white blood cells, skeletal muscle and the central nervous system.

In the retina there are two binding proteins specific to taurine. And, intracellular concentrations are higher in the retina than in any other region derived from the central nervous system. A deficiency state of taurine is often associated with an imbalance in intestinal flora. This condition, dysbiosis, is commonly called "leaky gut" and inhibits taurine absorption. Lowered levels of taurine may also be associated with cardiac arrhythmias, disorders of platelet formation, an overgrowth of candida, physical or emotional stress, a zinc deficiency, and excessive consumption of alcohol. Diabetes increases the retina's requirements for taurine. It is also important to note that the drugs chlorpromazine, a tranquilizer, and chloroquine, an anti-malarial/anti-inflammatory agent, inhibit the uptake of taurine and have been known to cause retinal damage with prolonged or excessive dosage.

Taurine helps protect cell membranes from oxidative attack. It helps transport nutrients across cell membranes, acts as a catalyst to retinal cells that remove cellular debris and assists in the elimination of potentially toxic substances. It is essential to the retinal pigment epithelium and the photoreceptor cells where it is found at levels ten times higher than the other free amino acids. Daily supplementation of 500 mg is advised.

How to Get All your Vitamins and Minerals

Taking a lot of pills every day, even for the most determined and motivated person, can be a problem. Multi vitamin and mineral pills solve this problem to some extent, but their ingredients may not be adequate for the special needs of those with macular degeneration. That is why I worked with a company to develop what I believe to be the most complete supplement for persons with macular degeneration. The formula I developed is the Macular Degeneration Nutritional Formula available from Nutritional Research LLC in Carson City, Nevada. This product contains 29 ingredients needed for the eye health, and is made from the freshest natural extracts. No artificial additives, preservatives, corn, wheat, yeast, soy, or dairy products are used in the manufacturing. Patients who have difficulty swallowing can open the capsule and mix the contents into fruit juice or sprinkle it on cereal.

At the end of this chapter is a list of the ingredients in the Macular Degeneration Nutritional Formula. You will notice that several ingredients are listed that I did not covered in this chapter. Be assured that they are very important for total eye health. For those patients who do not want to buy an extra product (i.e. Pure Focus), and wish to take all their nutrients from this formula, it contains baseline levels of lutein, vitamin E, and zeaxanthin, which will be described below.

Lutein and Zeaxanthin

In the first chapter I attempted to give you a picture of the physiology of the eye, and how macular degeneration affects the eye. I am now going to explain this in more detail, in order to help you understand some of the nutritional recommendations I will make in this and the following chapters. First of all, the complete name of the macula is the macula lutea. This means yellow spot, and it is a bright yellow spot, about one and a half millimeters in diameter in the center of the retina, which is about 20 mm in diameter itself. The macula is like a bull's eye that has the job of providing central vision and color vision.

The eye contains a pigment that serves the same purpose as melanin – to protect it from sun damage. It is called the xanthophyll pigment. Its two forms are lutein and zeaxanthin. These yellow pigments found in our food, are actually hidden in some green leaves, and are revealed when the leaves begin to turn yellow or orange. Perhaps you have seen a nice fresh bunch of kale turn yellow in your vegetable bin.

The job of these pigments is to absorb the ultra violet and visable blue rays of sunlight so that they do not burn the delicate tissues of the retina. While we are given a fairly good supply of them as children, most of us begin to lose xanthophyll pigments as early as our twenties or thirties. Daily consumption of leafy green vegetables, especially spinach, kale, mustard and collard greens, keeps our eyes supplied with xanthophyll pigments. Research has shown that eating food rich in the xanthophyll pigments immediately increases the amount measurable in your blood, and soon after, the amount seen in the macula of the eye. The amount in the macula is measured by macula pigment density. Pigment in the macula correlates to the health of the macula. Diminishing color vision occurs when the pigment in the macula becomes depleted. This is one of the early signs of macular degeneration.

Lutein and zeaxanthin are the names of the specific carotenes required by the macula to preserve thick pigment. Lutein and zeaxanthin have been found in abundance in just a few specific foods. These are, in the order of the amount of lutein and zeaxanthin they contain: Carotenoid content of selected vegetables (micrograms (mcg) container per 100 grams (g) portion.

Kale	21,900 mcg
Collard Greens	16,300 mcg
*Spinach – cooked	12,600 mcg
*Spinach – raw	10,200 mcg
Mustard Greens	9,900 mcg
Okra	6,800 mcg
Red Pepper	6,800 mcg
Romaine Lettuce	5,700 mcg
Endive	4,000 mcg
Cooked Broccoli	1,800 mcg
Green Peas	1,700 mcg
Pumpkin	1,500 mcg
Brussels Sprouts	1,300 mcg
Summer Squash	1,200 mcg

*Contains high amounts of oxalic acid.
Use in moderate amounts. Cook and/or add vinegar or fresh lemon juice to prevent osteoporosis or kid ney stones.

Better Nutrition Improves Your Results

11 Use Homeopathy and Chelation Therapy to Improve your Results

It is my sincere hope that by now you have obtained a Microcurrent Stimulation unit and are well acquainted with it. Even better, you have begun to use it on a regular basis and are beginning to experience moments of clearer vision and/or a gradual, steady improvement in your sight. I know this is possible because I have seen many of my patients achieve these results, and, of course, I was almost as delighted as they were, because my life's work is devoted to natural ways to treat vision problems.

It is because of this vocational interest, that I became thoroughly trained in the science and art of homeopathy. Twenty-five years ago, when I entered medical school, I had a burning desire to help people. Today, that is still my goal, but the way I go about it is the result of a long personal and professional journey.

I have always been competitive and like to engage in very demanding and rigorous sports. While training for the Hawaii Ironman Triathlon in 1988, a friend suggested I take a homeopathic remedy to help me cope with the muscle and joint pain of over-training. I was astonished at the results. My pain disappeared in a very short time, and there were no side effects from the remedy as there would have been if I had taken a prescription or an over-the-counter pain reliever. Being a scientist, I could not ignore what had happened to me, and I wanted to learn more about homeopathy. I soon discovered a world of experts and lectures where my learning could expand rapidly. Along the way I heard about the Hahnemann College of Homeopathy, located near San Francisco. I enrolled in a program of professional homeopathic studies. I found that homeopathy, like all complete systems of healing, was a very complex subject. Although it was difficult to add this study to an already full medical practice, I consider it very worthwhile. It has enabled me to help people in a way that is both natural and highly effective.

For my thesis in homeopathy, I decided to research how the early homeopaths treated eye disease in the 18th and 19th century. Because many of the old books have been preserved, I was able to uncover a wealth of information, and have done some pioneering work in bringing this work into prominence within the field. There is a long history of treating eye conditions with homeopathy. For about 70 years, from 1870 to 1940, the College of the New York Ophthalmic Hospital offered post graduate courses in homeopathic ophthalmology. During this period, there was one medical specialty society devoted to homeopathy and ophthalmology and two journals published in the US. From 1870 to 1916, twelve major works on the homeopathic treatment of eye diseases were published. Many cases were published in the literature of the time, showing improvement in a variety of eye diseases. These were all the more remarkable since there were no other treatments available at the time for serious eye disorders. Because this is still true with macular degeneration, homeopathy is a vitally important part of therapy for this condition.

The study of and research in homeopathy gave me a sound foundation for adding this therapy to my eye practice. The character of my practice has changed considerably. Now I can offer hope to my patients with macular degeneration, diabetic retinopathy, glaucoma, cataracts and eyestrain. Furthermore, they can take charge of their illness and begin to heal by making lifestyle changes as well as by using natural healing techniques. Introducing homeopathy, along with nutrition and other natural methods of healing into my practice has vastly increased my satisfaction in being a doctor. It has also brought hope and relief to many of my patients.

Since adding homeopathic treatment to my practice, I have treated many patients who have macular degeneration with homeopathy. The results have been highly satisfying to them as well as to me. I urge you to consider homeopathic treatment along with Microcurrent Stimulation. Homeopathy is also compatible with chelation. Doing all three treatments will provide a comprehensive healing experience as well as maximize your chance of reversing your eye disease.

179

What is Homeopathy?

Homeopathy is one of the most dynamic and easy-to-use methods of total healing. By total healing, I mean that homeopathy can heal your mental attitude, emotional state, as well as your physical disease. I have seen it work absolute wonders for my patients regardless of their eye condition. For those with macular degeneration, it offers hope for great improvement in vision as well as in transforming one's attitude about the condition. Patients with macular degeneration who have taken a homeopathic remedy not only notice improved vision but they report being calmer, more peaceful, less irritable, and able to enjoy the normal activities of life, fully. They no longer focus on how their condition limits them, but feel restored to a sense of gratitude for all that life offers.

Many scientists and other types of teachers speak of the connection between mind and body. Some names you may recognize include Deepak Chopra, Larry Dossey MD, Bernie Siegal MD, and Joan Borysenko PhD. All of these experts have proven, in their own way, that subtle and non-material aspects of our being, such as thoughts and feelings, have an impact on our physical state and well being. Conversely, they demonstrate that physical qualities such as blood sugar levels and muscular tension profoundly affect our thoughts and feelings. As our sense of well being and physical perception of ourselves improve, there is a corresponding improvement in our disease. Homeopathy helps the connection between mind and bodywork synergistically to bring about a rapid improvement in both.

Homeopathy is a natural system of healing based on the principle that 'like cures like.' This means that the symptoms of a disease resemble the symptoms that might be brought on in a healthy person who took the remedy under consideration. While this is the underlying principle of homeopathy, it does not tell us how it works. In fact, we don't know how it works.

Homeopathic remedies, in addition to matching the person's symptoms, are made from minute doses of the substance used to heal those symptoms. The doses are so tiny that, at some strength, the substance cannot even be detected in a chemical analysis of the remedy. And these strengths, called the high potencies, are the most powerful in their ability to heal! Some feel that homeopathy is a type of energy medicine, one that works on the non-material levels of the person. Others feel that we cannot measure the substance because our instruments are not that subtle yet. Regardless of how it works, the important thing for me and for you too is to know that it does work. Equally important is the fact that there are usually no side effects from homeopathic remedies. They do not accumulate in the body like ordinary medicine so there are no long-term adverse effects. However, one may have a permanent cure from as little as one dose of a remedy.

Homeopathic Remedies

Homeopathic remedies are made from plants, animals, and minerals. There are about 3000 remedies. The key to success in homeopathy is selecting the correct remedy. While it is true that about three dozen remedies cover a wide variety of illnesses and will help a large number of people, it is still important to consider all the remedies when prescribing for a case. Remedies come in two forms. The dry form, or pellets, consisting of small sugar pills taken by mouth under the tongue. This form is very easy and pleasant to take. Equally pleasant, but a little more complex is taking a liquid form of the remedy. These are prescribed by homeopaths, and, if you should need one, he or she will give you instructions. Unlike prescription or even over-the-counter drugs, remedies are taken for a short time only. In fact, you may only need one dose of a remedy to have a profound healing response. This is because of the way remedies work

Remedies come in a wide variety of strengths, called potencies. The remedies available in the health food stores are in the low to low-mid range in potency. Higher potencies, which are almost always needed to heal a serious chronic or degenerative condition, are available only by prescription through homeopaths. Although I do not suggest that you try to self treat your macular degeneration, I do suggest that you go to a health food store and look at the selection of homeopathic remedies. You will probably see several types of remedies. One type may be labeled according to a disease or conditions, such as arthritis, sinus or indigestion. These may be either tablets or tinctures which are liquid forms. They will contain a number of remedies, and, thus, are called combination remedies. I consider these somewhat useful for people to get acquainted with homeopathy, but they do not in any way represent the full power of homeopathy, and are not powerful enough to have any effect against macular degeneration.

Most likely you will also see some single remedies with unfamiliar names. These are likely to be packaged in small tubes. Inside are tiny white pellets. These are the most familiar and frequently used homeopathic remedies. People with some experience and knowledge of homeopathy use these to treat themselves, their families, and their pets. Although I strongly advise you to consult a skilled homeopathic practitioner to treat your macular degeneration, you may find these remedies useful for other conditions.

How do Remedies Work?

Homeopathic remedies work to stimulate your own vital force to heal your illness. Although they are taken in a form that resembles regular medicine, they are completely different. For example if you took antibiotics for a bacterial infection such as strep throat, the antibiotics would actually kill the germs that caused the infection. However, if you were to take a homeopathic remedy for that same condition, the remedy would stimulate your immune system to overcome the germs. And it would do this without causing any side effects, whatsoever.

Another way remedies differ from regular medicine is in their timing. Many prescription drugs need to accumulate in your system before they can affect it. Anti-depressants are one example. A person often needs to take an anti-depressant for several weeks before it has any effect. In homeopathy, there is no such thing as a cumulative effect. You can take one dose of a remedy and have an immediate effect. Or you can take one dose and have an effect several days or weeks later without taking any more doses. This is because the remedy works deeply in your system to mobilize your own healing forces. People who have been seriously ill and/or ill for a long time may require a longer period before they notice a response to a remedy. They may also require a repeated dose in a few months' time. A homeopath will carefully observe your response to the remedy that is prescribed and determine the potency and frequency of repetition.

The Power of Homeopathy

One of the reasons why I have dedicated so much of my life and my practice to homeopathy is because of its power. It can cure disease states at every level of seriousness. For example, it is very effective in what we call 'acute' illness. This means short-term intense diseases like flu, fever, pneumonia, and some injuries. It is also highly effective in curing chronic illness such as asthma, arthritis, lupus, and eye conditions. It can help where conventional medicine has nothing to offer besides powerful, potentially destructive medications. With a condition like macular degeneration, where conventional medicine has no cure or even effective treatment, homeopathy is a wonderful resource. It is also excellent at resolving deep emotional states such as anxiety, unexpressed or lingering grief, and depression. Mental/emotional disorders like panic attacks and attention deficit disorder respond beautifully. Even when people have terminal illness and organ changes that make it impossible for them to recover, homeopathy can relieve their pain as well as bring peace to their final days.

The Discovery of Homeopathy

You may be wondering where this powerful healing system originated. You may also be wondering why it is not used more often and accepted as part of standard medicine. Samuel Hahnemann (1755-1843) was born in Germany and is considered the father of homeopathy. While homeopathy is based upon some ancient systems of healing as well as folk knowledge and herbal medicine, many aspects of it are entirely his original contribution. The idea of using a minute dose of medicine was never applied so effectively or systematically before Hahnemann. Some of the ideas in homeopathy are used in regular medicine. One concept that uses the principle of minute dose and like cures like is in immunization. Currently, the idea of using fractional or small doses of chemotherapy in place of the massive doses is becoming an accepted part of medical practice.

Use Homeopathy and Chelation Therapy

Homeopathy, once a very popular form of medicine, had its demise in the US as a result of the growth of the pharmaceutical companies. There is virtually no opportunity to make large profits in the manufacture of homeopathic remedies. Also, homeopathy does not lend itself to standardized research for a number of reasons. So, with the growth in power of conventional medicine, homeopathy went underground in the US until its rebirth about twenty-five years ago. There are now many fine training programs operating in the US as well as abroad and the number of qualified homeopaths is increasing yearly. More and more research is being done to demonstrate the effectiveness of remedies. But perhaps the most important reason for the resurgence of homeopathy is the groundswell of recognition of its usefulness in treating chronic conditions that are virtually unresponsive to the drugs of conventional medicine. I predict that economics will have an increasing role in reviving homeopathy when managed care organizations begin to see the results it produces for a fraction of the cost of regular prescriptions. And, when they factor in the long term gains in health status, meaning that those treated homeopathically enjoy a higher level of health in general, they are bound to include it in their treatment mix.

Choosing a Homeopath

Many people purport to practice homeopathy, but, in my opinion, only some of these people are qualified to do so. I am going to give you guidelines to use in selecting a homeopath if you decide to pursue this type of treatment. Some homeopaths are MDs; some are chiropractors, naturopaths or acupuncturists. Some are homeopaths who are not trained in any other form of medicine. Ideally, what you should look for is a classically trained homeopath who is certified by the Council for Homeopathic Certification and uses the letters CCH after their name, or one who is certified by the American Homeopathic Association and uses the letters DHt after their name. These individuals have passed a test that demonstrates the high level of their competence. They have also met rigorous standards with respect to their education. There are individuals who are highly skilled homeopaths who have not taken these certification tests, however.

The National Center for Homeopathy maintains a list of practicing homeopaths throughout the US. This organization makes no claims about the competence of those it lists, but is a good place to start if you do not know how to find a homeopath in your area. Finally you can visit the website of the Hahnemann College of Homeopathy which maintains a list of its graduates. I can vouch for the quality of their training since that is where I received mine.

A Visit to a Homeopath

A visit to a homeopath is quite different than an appointment with a regular doctor. First of all, the homeopath will be interested in many things about you that an ordinary doctor would ignore. Homeopaths consider the way that you think, feel, look, as well as the effects of your particular illness. To a homeopath, everything about a person expresses who they are and what medicine they might need. For example, your tendency to be warm or chilly as well as food preferences are important in understanding your case. Even if a homeopath saw three people with macular degeneration in one day, they would focus on the unique aspects of each person's situation. One person might be quite passive in accepting their diagnosis while another might be very anxious. One person might fear that their eye condition was a sign of other underlying disease, while another might feel grateful that they had only an eye condition. Similarly, one person might have insomnia or anxiety at night while another sleeps soundly but awakens with a headache almost every day. All of these distinctions would be important to the homeopath. Along with these characteristics, the homeopath might ask about your childhood and your dreams.

Many people report that their visit to a homeopath is one of their most enjoyable experiences. The visit usually takes from one to two hours and is conducted in a relaxing way. The homeopath's focus is completely on the client and on anything he or she wants to discuss.

There is no pressure to discuss things that make the client uncomfortable.

Shortly after the visit, the homeopath will prescribe a remedy and will tell the client how to obtain it. The next appointment will probably be in four to six weeks. At that time the homeopath will assess how well the remedy has worked. He or she may or may not make a new prescription at that time. In terms of expectations, it is important for patients to know that long term chronic conditions may take a while to resolve fully. A rule of thumb is that a month is required to heal for each year of the disease. However, the remedy begins to work deeply as soon as it is taken, and the person's underlying state is being strengthened.

Homeopathy and Microcurrent Stimulation

There is absolutely no conflict between using Microcurrent Stimulation and homeopathy at the same time. If your homeopath wonders about this, show this book to him or her. Remember, by the time your macular degeneration manifests symptomatically, you probably have a fair amount of disease tendencies manifesting in different organs and systems, even if you do not have symptoms of the diseases. This is another reason to move ahead at full speed and include as many natural ways to heal as you can. When your condition has improved, it will not matter to you which technique was most beneficial. Take advantage of the synergy of natural healing. Read on to learn about yet another fantastic way to heal yourself of many degenerative conditions as well as macular degeneration.

Chelation Therapy: Remove Toxic Metals and Improve Blood Flow

Chelation Therapy, like Microcurrent Stimulation and Homeopathy requires your own natural vital force in order to work well. These three therapies are not drugs that you can take or operations you can undergo where you have no active part in your healing. On the contrary, for these methods to work as well as they can, you must be in the best possible health. With the chapter on diet and supplements, I have given you some powerful tools to improve your underlying state of health. With optimal health, you can handle your macular degeneration much better on the emotional level and cope with vision changes and mobility issues much more successfully while you are waiting for improved vision. With Microcurrent Stimulation underway and enjoying a vastly improved nutritional program, you are ready to add Chelation Therapy to your regimen.

Although you may never have heard of chelation, it has been employed by doctors in this country since about 1950, following its development in Germany in 1938. This is a treatment normally used by doctors to treat lead poisoning and even venomous snakebites. In the early years of its use, it was discovered that chelation improved the heart disease of those who underwent it for other purposes. This prompted a number of physicians to begin using it for this purpose alone. It has been proven to flush plaque and toxic metals from bloodstream. For many, many individuals it has been an alternative to heart or vascular surgery.

In chelation therapy, about three grams of a chemical called ethyl-diamine- tetra-acetic acid (EDTA) is used for each treatment. Although EDTA has been approved to treat lead poisoning and some other conditions, it has not been approved for use in treating heart and vascular conditions. This does not mean that it is harmful or ineffective in these instances. Many drugs and devices are used in this way in the medical field. The devices used for Microcurrent Stimulation are an example. When doctors use chelation for purposes other than lead poisoning, they are using an approved substance, the synthetic amino acid EDTA in a discretionary way. This is done frequently in medicine. One example familiar to us all is the use of aspirin, which is approved for the treatment of pain. However, physicians routinely recommend it to persons with cardiovascular disease as a blood thinner.

A Chelation Treatment Session

A chelation treatment requires a visit to a doctor's office where a substance is infused into your veins through an IV for the purpose of helping your body rid itself of toxic heavy metals and excess minerals. Chelation requires a course of treatment of several sessions per week for several weeks or months. It is recommended that patients undergo 30 chelation treatments in order to obtain the optimum effect, and follow these with a maintenance treatment once a month. Each session lasts two to four hours. The frequency of the treatments depends on the severity of the condition and the way that the body is handling the excretion of the minerals. During the course of treatment, the doctor will monitor the health of your kidneys as well as other organs to ensure that no undue stress is placed on the body. There is almost no discomfort with chelation and the side effects, which are rare, are very minimal. Chelation patients are instructed in proper diet, stress management, and exercises to support their overall recovery.

How to Find a Doctor for Chelation

Chelation is administered by medical doctors (MDs) and Doctors of Osteopathy (DOs) who have been specially trained and are accredited by the American College for the Advancement of Medicine (ACAM). This organization was founded in 1973 as a medical society to educate and update physicians on the latest in preventive and nutritional advances against disease. Although there may be other health practitioners who use chelation, I would strongly recommend that you work only with a doctor who is a member of ACAM. The ACAM maintains a list of doctors who are trained and certified to administer chelation therapy. The actual certification is done by the American Board of Chelation Therapy. This group monitors the preparation for this recognized medical subspecialty. It is important for you to work with such an individual. This means that he or she knows how to match the dose of EDTA to your particular condition and to monitor your overall health during the course of treatment.

Chelation has been used very successfully to treat cardiovascular disease, diabetes, diabetic arterial disease, decreased mental functioning, intermittent claudication (leg pain on exercise), and a number of other conditions. Eye conditions such as glaucoma and cataract have responded to chelation therapy. It has also been used to reverse macular degeneration since macular degeneration is caused, at least in part, by the blockage in the choroid capillaries, which deliver blood to the macula.

In 1994, the *Journal of the Advancement of Medicine* published a case where a 59-year old woman with macular degeneration used nutrition along with chelation for her condition. After undergoing the recommended series of chelation treatments, her vision improved to 20/25 in one eye and 20/20 in the other. Her central vision was greatly enhanced. One year later, her vision improvement remained.

How Chelation Works

The word "chelation" is taken from the Greek work *chele,* meaning claw. This describes the way the molecules of the chelating agent grab onto the molecules of heavy metal, such as lead, iron, and copper, in the body and moves them to the kidneys, via the bloodstream, for excretion. The process of chelation also binds calcium, which is known, when it is present in cells in excessive amounts, to interfere with arterial health. Calcium is responsible for the build-up of plaque that causes blockages in the blood vessels. None of the calcium chelated and released during chelation is the calcium from bones and teeth. Chelation lowers serum ionized calcium which decreases clotting, reduces spasm and softens "hardening" of the arteries. A further benefit to overall health is that EDTA reduces the LDL cholesterol (the so-called 'bad' cholesterol) content in the liver and the plaque formed in the arteries.

Despite its success, scientists do not know for certain how chelation works. One theory is that it reduces free radicals. As I explained in the chapter on nutrition, free radicals are the harmful by-products of metabolic processes. Since heavy metals cause an increased production of free radicals, reducing them in the body reduces the numbers of free radicals. Yet another understanding of how chelation works focuses on the relationship between calcium and magnesium as intracellular and intercellular components. As excess calcium is bound in the bloodstream, the calcium/magnesium balance is favorably affected. This results in a great improvement in arterial health.

Chelation and The Medical Profession

Unfortunately the medical profession does not recognize chelation therapy as an accepted treatment. Beyond this, there are physicians who erroneously believe that it is harmful, or, at best, not useful. They will surely discourage their patients from using it. I want to emphasize that, in the more than 40 years it has been used in this country, only two deaths have occurred that can be attributed to chelation. These occurred in the nineteen fifties, when there was insufficient knowledge about drug dosage and administration. Conventional medicine has made much of these two deaths while they conveniently ignore the 100,000 deaths each year from prescription drugs. I consider this to be a very safe treatment when performed by a well-trained physician.

When you are up against skepticism and downright ignorance from the medical profession, you have a unique opportunity. This is the time for you to become your strongest advocate for the recovery of your vision as well as your overall health. Why wait and let time pass while your vision deteriorates when there are techniques that can be helpful? Medical science is notoriously slow to recognize and approve methods that have arisen from outside the pharmaceutical/medical technology fields. Unfortunately, these giant profit-making businesses have quite a grip on research and innovation in medicine. Doctors who fail to do their own research on chelation therapy are not in a position to evaluate it. You may need to do this for yourself. A good starting point is the information you can request from the ACAM. The books written by Dr. Morton Walker are also a valuable resource in learning about chelation therapy from both a scientific as well as case study perspective.

Use Homeopathy and Chelation Therapy

I have outlined two additional therapies for you to consider in reversing your macular degeneration. Please think about them seriously. Some factors to consider are the convenience of finding a practitioner of the therapy you choose as well as price and time commitment. Chelation is arguably the most expensive of the therapies but is invaluable if you have circulatory disorders along with macular degeneration. Homeopathy is generally not very expensive, but you may not be able to find a qualified practitioner. This brings us back to the wonderful availability of Microcurrent Stimulation. While you think about homeopathy and chelation, you can order your unit and get started.

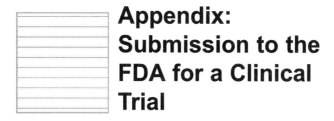

Appendix: Submission to the FDA for a Clinical Trial

Written, except as otherwise noted, by Joel Rossen DVM

Introduction

Age-related Macular Degeneration (ARMD) and cataracts are the major causes of visual impairment and blindness in the United States in persons over 55 years of age. ARMD damages the retinal tissue in the macular area causing fine pigmentary stippling, retinal pigment epithelium changes, and the development of drusen. Drusen usually occur in a mirror pattern in both eyes, but not necessarily. As you will read below, drusen is typically consists of a buildup of proteinaceous waste materials.

Appendix: Study Submitted to FDA

ARMD can be wet (exudative) or dry (non-exudative). The dry type is characterized initially by either normal acuity or only a moderate acuity loss that commonly progresses to a severe acuity loss. The wet type may progress to rapid and severe vision loss. At the present time there is no recognized therapy for the dry type of ARMD and the common treatment for the wet type, which must be done within 24 hours of a bleed, is laser coagulation and obliteration of the offending vessels. The percentage of patients who benefit from this laser therapy is estimated at about 4%.[1]

With dry ARMD, yellow-white deposits called drusen accumulate in the retinal pigment epithelium (RPE) tissue beneath the macula. Drusen deposits are composed of waste products from photoreceptor cells. These waste products are sometimes called discs. For reasons few people understand, RPE tissue can lose its ability to process waste. As a result, drusen deposits accumulate in the RPE. Drusen deposits are typically present in patients with dry ARMD.

The drusen deposits are thought to interfere with the function of photoreceptors in the macula, causing progressive degeneration of these cells. I do not believe that drusen are actually a cause of loss of VA, they are an effect of loss of energetic vitality. I believe that the deficient cellular housekeeping efficiency, which is directly proportional to the decrease in the intracellular concentration of ATP, is responsible for the buildup of drusen. Although drusen may block light transfer and obstruct the cell's functions, including the regeneration of rhodopsin, I believe that the drusen is a symptom of a more elemental dysfunction.

While there is a tendency for drusen to be blamed for the progressive loss of vision, drusen deposits can, however, be present in the retina without vision loss. It is very important to keep this in mind. Some patients with large deposits of drusen have normal visual acuity. If normal retinal reception and image transmission is sometimes possible in a retina when high concentrations of drusen are present, then even if drusen can be implicated in the loss of visual function, **there MUST be at least one other factor** which accounts for the loss of vision.

The point of minimum effort for re-establishment or enhancement of vision may lie outside the drusen mechanism. It might be theoretically possible for the drusen to stay and for the vision be re-established, enhanced, or at least maintained. If there is actually another metabolic/biological component that is the pin upon which hinges the vision function, then we must identify and address that component.

Some literature states that optic nerve head drusen (hyaline bodies), represent calcific and proteinaceous materials that are confined anterior to the lamina cribrosa within the optic nerve head. These calcium deposits are believed to be derived from axonal debris that results from alterations in axoplasmic flow. Optic nerve heads with drusen are small in size with an elevated appearance and irregular margins.

Other sources state that the drusen is a complex of up to 11 different hyaline (protein) molecules and these sources do not address a calcium component.[2] CMSD studies indicate that drusen are similar in molecular composition to plaques and deposits in other age-related diseases such as Alzheimer's disease and atherosclerosis.

The presence of optic nerve head drusen appears to cause visual field defects and may alter the vascular supply to the optic nerve head. Progressive damage is possible and can result in ischemic optic neuropathy. (I do not agree that the drusen is necessarily causative of visual field defect. Author)

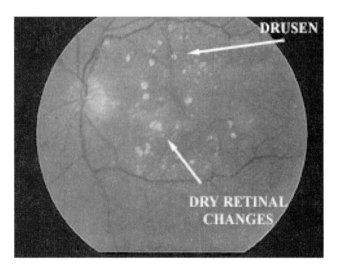

Hypotheses

Hypothesis: Underlying the symptoms normally seen in patients diagnosed with ARMD is a more fundamen-

tal and elemental metabolic imbalance. A normal part of aging is the loss of efficiency of the cellular energy management systems. This is due, at least in part, to a decrease in mitochondrial function. Insufficient mitochondrial output of ATP naturally leads to low concentrations of intracellular ATP. The decrease in mitochondrial function results from free radical damage and mutation of mtDNA (mitochondrial DNA).

ARMD is considered to be a retinal disease. I propose that this disease is much more complex than simply being a disease of the retina. I believe it is part of an age related, energy processing syndrome. I also propose that those very complexities of vision, that is, its dependence on ATP availability, provide the inherent keys that enigmatically simplify the treatment of the disease.

MicroCurrent has been shown to increase intracellular concentrations of ATP.[3] The complete mechanism by which this occurs is unknown. If the aging process is truly characterized by ATP deficiencies and ARMD is truly a disease of aging, then the stimulation of ATP production could be the reason that microcurrent can aid in the control of the degeneration associated with ARMD.

Protein synthesis is enhanced by microcurrent stimulation. So is the cell's ability to absorb nutrients and to produce ATP. Currents in the neighborhood of 500 microAmps have been shown to increase APT concentrations up to 500%.[4] Electrical resistance of the Schwann cell sheaths is decreased by establishing an increased electrical charge on the cells and a significant amount of information is processed and transmitted, not via the traditional waves of depolarization of the cell membrane, but also via an analog current carried by the myelin sheaths.[5]

What is an increase in visual acuity? It is an increase in the eye's ability to deliver a signal or series of signals to the brain, which are perceived a higher resolution image?

And how do you get more products (signal) to market (perception)? ANSWER: Increase the amount of information being transmitted and increase the bandwidth (eliminate the transmission bottlenecks).

Hypotheses to be tested:

1.) Stimulating the eyes with Microcurrent will slow, stop, and in some cases, to some degree, reverse the symptoms of Age Related Macular Degeneration.

2.) Stimulating the eyes with microcurrent in the presence of nutritional supplementation, specifically a combination of nutrients designed to decrease the oxidative destruction of the mitochondria and ATP synthase, will slow, stop, and in some cases, to some degree, reverse the symptoms of Age Related Macular Degeneration.

3.) Stimulation of the eyes with Microcurrent causes a retinal stimulation. The patient sees flashing when

202

the eye is stimulated. A group of patients who receive a placebo or sham treatment consisting of a red flashing light which simulates the flashing phenomenon observed when the eyes are stimulated with electricity will show less improvement than the group receiving the real stimulation.

Mitochondria and Aging

Of the many different theories of aging, they all have the second law of thermodynamics in common. "The universe constantly changes so as to become more disordered".

The ATP Synthesizing Enzymes of the Mitochondria

ATP synthesizing enzymes have been shown to suffer oxidative damage that effects the efficiency of ATP production (Shigenaga, '94, p.10775). Research has shown "age related changes of the mitochondrial energy metabolism in rat liver and heart, indicating a decrease of the ATP synthase activity, and accompanied by a decrease of the amount of beta subunit" of the F0F1 ATPase.[6] (Kroll, '96, p.57).

Guerrieri Et. Al, [7] claim to have shown functional and structural differences of the mitochondrial F0F1 ATP synthase complex in the hearts of aged rats (24 months old) when compared to young rats (3 months old). They relate this to the alteration of cellular energy metabolism observed in aged animals. The accumulation of free radicals and the decrease of antioxidant systems could cause alteration of the oxidative phosphorylation mechanism" This does not conflict with the mitochondrial DNA mutation theory because the beta subunit of ATP synthase is encoded by nuclear DNA.

Mutation and Damage to Mitochondrial DNA

The mitochondrial DNA (mtDNA), which resembles the circular bacterial DNA, only codes for about thirteen of the proteins that are found in the electron transport chain. The majority of the proteins, approximately sixty, are encoded from nuclear DNA. Both mtDNA and nuclear DNA are susceptible to mutations by oxygen free radicals. This can cause death or dysfunction of the mitochondria and eventual cell death by interfering with oxidative phosphorylation. Frequencies of mutations differ between mtDNA and nuclear DNA.

The occurrences of mtDNA mutations are much higher than nuclear DNA mutations. The levels of oxidative damage to mtDNA range from ten to seventeen times that in nuclear DNA, depending on the part of the body sampled. Shigenaga has been proposed that this is due to the mitochondrial association with oxygen.[8]

Not only do mitochondria have a greater rate of mutation but they also lack DNA repair mechanisms. This means that through mitotic divisions, mitochondrial DNA mutations are likely to accumulate with age.[9] (Stephenson, '96, p.1532).

Mitochondrial Lipid Membranes and Antioxidants

Lipid membranes are also susceptible to oxidative damage over time. The fluidity of cellular and mitochondrial membranes decreases with age due in part to the changes in membrane compositions and lipid peroxidation. A diphosphatidyl glycerol derivative in the mitochondria, called cardiolipin, performs many important roles in membrane structure and function. Among them, cardiolipin contributes to the control of permeability of the inner mitochondrial membrane to small molecules and helps maintains the electrochemical proton gradient. The sensitivity to oxidation increases with age and the amount of this valuable membrane compound supposedly decreases with age. This is paralleled by a decrease of the inner membrane surface area, and increased fragility of the mitochondria (Shigenaga, '94, p.10774-5).

A decrease in inner membrane surface decreases the cells' abilities to synthesize. Increased mitochondrial fragility will increase mitochondrial attrition. Both cases decrease ATP concentrations in the cells.

Glutathione (GSH), an intracellular antioxidant agent, has been shown to protect the oxidative phosphorylation mechanisms from the ravaging effects of free radicals. This is done by the binding of the GSH molecule to the ATP synthase complex which somehow protects them from unwanted oxidation.

Antioxidants which can be found in foods include

ascorbate, tocopherol, and carotenoids. Evidence indicates that protection from aging ailments such as cancer, cardiovascular disease, and brain dysfunction can be avoided or at least minimized by dietary intake of fruits and vegetables that are high in antioxidants (Shigenaga, '94,p.10771). Melatonin, a new face on the antioxidant scene, is a primary pineal hormone that acts as an hydroxyl (OH-) scavenger (Yu and Yang, '96, p.7,9).[10]

Mitochondria Section Conclusion

Since the mitochondria are the main energy producers of organisms, if they are not functioning properly diseases usually result. The coordinated interactions between antioxidants, ATP synthase, DNA, and the free radicals are in a delicate balance through the early portion of life and gradually go out of balance, causing disease by degradation of the mitochondria. This is what we see as the phenotype of aging.

The Relationship Between ATP, Mitochondrial Function, and Vision

I believe that there are a number of metabolic factors that participate in the ARMD complex. The medical community generally accepts some of these and some not. It is possible that the complex of symptoms which, in tandem, define the ARMD syndrome, are simply a set of symptoms which are actually related because they are all sequellae of the body's deteriorating energy subsystem.

206

These five functions are all possible ways in which the MicroStim® could conceivably affect visual acuity in ARMD patients.

1.) Re-synthesizing visual purple and rhodopsin after light reception and transmission has taken place. How quickly the visual purple and rhodopsin can be re-synthesized after they breakdown and send or attempt to send a signal to the brain will affect light sensing efficiency.

2.) Rebuilding the intracellular ATP concentration after the ATP has been depleted. After a nerve fires (depolarizes) ATP is used to re-establish neurological cell membrane potential. ATP is used to supply the energy that is needed when the cell removes metabolic waste and imports fresh metabolites using the active transport mechanism.

3.) Re-polarization of the optic nerves. Adequate intracellular concentrations of ATP, which is produced in the Mitochondria, are essential for the optic nerve to transfer information to the brain after its fibers have been stimulated by the rods or cones. This [ATP] concentration will affect the functioning of the sodium pump and hence, affect the cell's ability to re-polarize (re-polarization efficiency). More specifically, a completely re-polarized neuron will have a cell membrane potential of about –85 milliVolts. When an action potential traverses the neuron, the cell membrane potential is reduced along the cell membrane. This reduction of the cell's polarization, which occurs as a wave of de-polarization, is the action potential. Hence, for the neuron to fire again, the cell membrane potential must be re-established.

4.) Possible genetic links that decrease energy efficiency and cause retinal disease by adversely affecting the body's ability to synthesize ATP could provide a clue to ARMD treatment. Strengthening the process of ATP synthesis could conceivably abort the degeneration prior to the point that the genetic defect works its damage.

5.) Cellular waste management: Loss of the ability to process waste materials and re-polarize is a common finding in aged and ATP deficient cells in all parts of the body.

It is possible that a technology that was capable of increasing cellular ATP concentration, specifically in the area of the eyes, could provide the means to achieve each of the 5 goals above.

ATP - Nature's Energy Store

All living things, plants and animals, require a continual supply of energy in order to function. The energy is used for all the processes that keep the organism alive. Some of these processes occur continually, such as the metabolism of foods, the synthesis of large, biologically important molecules, e.g. proteins and DNA, and the transport of molecules and ions throughout the organism. Other processes occur only at certain times, such as muscle contraction and other cellular movements. Animals obtain their energy by oxidation of foods, plants do so by trapping the sunlight using chlorophyll. However, before the energy can be used, it is first transformed into a form that the organism can handle easily. This special carrier of energy is the molecule adenosine triphosphate, or ATP.

ATP Metabolism and Synthesis

The Different Metabolic Effects of Standard Millicurrent TENS v.s. MicroCurrent.

Even though, up to now, both MicroCurrent and TENS devices have tended to be classified as substantially equivalent to pre-amendment TENS devices, there appears to be a very elemental divergence between the biological effects of the two technologies. While at the upper end of the TENS current spectrum, the electrical stimulation can block the neurological transmission of pain signals, there appears to be a divergence of the effects at the lower end, the MicroCurrent end.

Research by Cheng ET AL[11], demonstrated a very significant difference between the types of electrical stimulators known as TENS devices and those classified as MicroCurrent devices. He demonstrated that currents in the range of about 200-750 microAmps tended to increase ATP concentrations in cells, while currents above 1 milliAmp tended to lower intracellular ATP concentrations.

ATP Structure

ATP has three main parts: A ribose sugar, adenine, and a triphosphate group. The three phosphates are linked together by two high-energy bonds. When the high-energy bonds are broken, energy is released from the ATP molecule. Usually, only one of the bonds is broken when the ATP is used by the body for energy.

The ATP molecule is composed of three components. At the center is a sugar molecule, ribose (the same sugar that forms the basis of DNA). Attached to one side of this is a base (a group consisting of linked rings of carbon and nitrogen atoms); in this case the base is adenine. The other side of the sugar is attached to a string of 3 phosphate groups. These phosphates are the keys to the activity of ATP. The three phosphates are linked together by high-energy bonds. When the high-energy bonds are broken, energy is released from the ATP molecule.

ATP Molecule

ATP Metabolism

ATP is adenosine triphosphate. It is synthesized in the mitochondria by the process that is known as the Kreb's cycle, the sequence of reactions in the mitochondria that complete the oxidation of glucose in respiration. This process of cellular respiration uses oxygen and glucose and releases CO_2 as a byproduct. This process uses the enzyme, ATP synthase, to combine phosphate radical with ADP (adenosine diphosphate) plus electrons (it is an endothermic reaction) supplied by the breakdown of pyruvate and glucose to create a relatively unstable, high-energy molecule called ATP. It is the high energy and the instability of this molecule that makes it valuable and useful.

ATP works by losing the endmost phosphate group when instructed to do so by an enzyme. This reaction releases a lot of energy, 7 caalories per gram, which the organism can then use to build proteins, contact muscles, etc. The reaction product is adenosine diphosphate (ADP), and the phosphate group either ends up as orthophosphate (HPO4) or attached to another molecule (e.g. an alcohol). Even more energy can be extracted by removing a second phosphate group to produce adenosine monophosphate (AMP). This event is less common.

When the organism is resting and energy is not immediately needed, the reverse reaction takes place and the phosphate group is reattached to the molecule using energy obtained from food or sunlight. Thus the ATP molecule acts as a chemical 'battery', storing energy when it is not needed, but able to release it instantly when the organism requires it.

The body must constantly generate ATP. A male body uses 8000 grams of ATP per hour. A male body can only hold 100 grams of ATP at a time. ATP can release 14 calories per gram, but this requires breaking both phosphate bonds. Usually only one phosphate bond is broken, hence 7 calories of energy release per gram is the norm. It is crucial that the system which produces ATP be maintained for optimal performance because the equivalent of all the ATP in the body must be replaced 80 times per hour (every 45 seconds).

The Kreb's cycle is the respiratory cycle that is responsible for cell respiration, the manufacture of ATP, and the production of the waste product, CO_2. The main function of the mitochondria is the oxidation of the pyruvate derived from glycolysis and related processes to produce the ATP required to perform the cellular work. Free radicals, a type of highly reactive, destructive molecules, are a byproduct of this process and may be implicated in the aging process.

A Kmown Genetic Link between ATP and Retinal Function

It is possible that ATP metabolism is one of the significant keys that may unlock the secrets of ARMD treatment. ATP Synthase, aka ATPase, is an enzzyme which catalyzes the synthesis of ATP. A genetic defect in the ATPase 6 gene has been implicated in the disease Retinitis Rigmentosa (RP). RP has similarities to ARMD, not the least of which is that RP is a type of progressive retinal degeneration.

The mitochondrial genome (mtDNA) in humans is contained on a single circular chromosome 16,569 basepairs around, and each mitochondrion contains 5 to 10 copies of the mitochondrial chromosome. There are several essential genes in mtDNA that are involved in replication and translation, along with some genes that are crucial for the machinery that converts metabolic energy into ATP. These include NADH dehydrogenase, cytochrome c oxidase, ubiquinol/cytochrome c oxidoreductase, and ATP synthase, as well as the genes for unique Ribosomal RNA and Transfer RNA particles that are required for translating these genes into proteins.

There are specific diseases associated with mutations in some of these genes. Below is one of the affected genes and the disease which arises from its mutation.

Mutation of the ATP synthase gene:

Myoclonic Epilepsy and Ragged Red Fiber disease, MERRF, involves mutation of the ATPase 8 gene. While Neurogenic muscle weakness, Ataxia, and **Retinitis Pigmentosum (RP),** NARP, results from mutations in the ATPase 6 gene

RP is a genetically linked dysfunction of the retina and is related to mutation of the ATP Synthase Gene 6[12].[1314]

The Role of ATP in The Active Transport Mechanism

ATP increases the cell's ability to re-polarize because it provides the fuel that powers the Active Transport Mechanism.

Active Transport

Active transport requires the expenditure of energy to transport the molecule from one side of the membrane to the other, but active transport is the only type of transport that can actually take molecules up their concentration gradient as well as down.

Similarly to facilitated transport, active transport is limited by the number of protein transporters present.

We are interested in two general categories of active transport, primary and secondary. Primary active transport involves using energy (usually through ATP hydrolysis) at the membrane protein itself to cause a conformational change that results in the transport of the molecule through the protein. The most well-known example of this is the Na+ K+ pump. The Na+ K+ pump is an antiport, it transports K+ into the cell and Na+ out of the cell at the same time, with the expenditure of ATP.

Secondary active transport involves using energy to establish a gradient across the cell membrane, and then utilizing that gradient to transport a molecule of interest up its concentration gradient. An example of this mechanism is as follows: E. coli establishes a proton (H+) gradient across the cell membrane by using energy to pump protons out of the cell. Then those protons are coupled to lactose at the lactose permease transmembrane protein. The lactose permease uses the energy of the proton moving down its concentration gradient to transport lactose into the cell. This coupled transport in the same direction across the cell membrane is known as a symport. E. coli uses similar proton driven symports to transport ribose, arabinose, and several amino acids.

The Na+ -glucose secondary transport mechanism

Another secondary active transport system uses the Na+-K+ pump as the first step, generating a strong

Na+ gradient across the cell membrane. Then the glu-cose-Na+ symport protein uses that Na+ gradient to trans-port glucose into the cell.

This system is used in a novel way in human gut epithelial cells. These cells take in glucose and Na+ from the intestines and transport them through to the blood stream using the concerted actions of Na+-glucose symports, glucose permeases (a glucose facilitated dif-fusion protein), and Na+-K+ pumps. Note that the epi-thelial cells are joined together by tight junctions to pre-vent anything from leaking through from the intestines to the blood stream without first being filtered by the epithelial cells.

Aging cells often experience a decrease in ATP concentration and then lose their ability to efficiently pro-cess metabolic waste. It is this deficiency which causes each of the active mechanisms to falter and causes the primary ATM (active transport mechanism) to malfunc-tion.

What else does the ATP and the active trans-port mechanism do?

Let's talk about neurological signal transmission because this is the focus of my understanding of why some retinas, even though infested with drusen, still func-tion to allow the complete transmission of vision signal to the brain. There are at least two very important events that occur when a nerve sends a signal. One event is analog and the other is digital. Both events are required for complete and accurate information process-ing/ signal transmission.

When a nerve fires, a wave of depolarization moves along its body towards the next synapse. This wave is called an action potential. A polarized nerve cell is in a ready state, ready to fire, ready to de-polarize. A polarized cell has an abundance of sodium (Na^+) ions external to the cell membrane and an abundance of potassium (K^+) ions on the intra-cellular membrane.

De-polarization is characterized by the sudden movement of Na^+ into the cell in exchange for K^+, which moves out of the cell. Although the nerve cell does not completely depolarize, its state of readiness is reduced. As a cell is further and further de-polarized, it response ability is further and further compromised.

In order for the nerve cell to reach its full potential,, both literally and figuratively, its membrane must be re-polarized. The process by which the cell is re-po-larized uses the energy which is provided by the break-down of ATP. This process depletes ATP stores.

Re-polarization of the cell is an 'uphill' battle. Both sodium and potassium ions must be transported against their potential gradients. When a solute needs to move from an area of lower to an area of higher concentration, normal laws of diffusion can not compensate. The solute calls on a Protein "buddy" for help across the membrane. The energy used to fuel this transportation comes from ATP, a chemical energy. It is often necessary for these solutes to be transported to the areas of higher concen-

217

tration for the cell to function.

The mechanism by which ions are moved against a concentration gradient is called the Active Transport Mechanism (ATM). The ATM is an electrochemical reaction that occurs at the cell membrane. This process is the mechanism by which metabolic waste and excess Na^+ are actively removed from the cell and glucose and K^+ are moved into the cell's interior.

Re-polarization and Cellular Housekeeping

How does the cell rid itself of metabolic waste and bring in fresh metabolic substrate (glucose)?

To a great extent, ATP is responsible for the most important cellular metabolic functions. It is often called the cell's currency. At the cell membrane, ATP is broken down when activated by the enzymes present at the membrane. These enzymes catalyze ATP to break down to ADP (Adenosine diphosphate) and Phosphate radical, and release electrons. At this point the freed electrons provide the energy to combine certain proteins with the metabolic waste materials which are the breakdown products of cellular metabolism. **In the retina, this includes the protein wastes from the breakdown of retinal cellular pigments (discs).**

This electromolecular change causes the metabolic waste to become differentially permeable in material that forms the cell membrane. What this means is that these waste products suddenly are imbued with the ability to dissolve into the cell membrane, but only in one direction, out. (Hence, the meaning of differentially permeable). The direction of permeability may have electronic/magnetic polarity as one of the factors affecting the direction of permeability. There is also an effect at the cell membrane that is the result of an excess of protons, which creates an ion pump that actively removes unneeded molecular waste, such as protein byproducts, from the cell.

Once out of the cell, the metabolic waste products are released into the bloodstream. A similar reaction occurs with metabolic substrate (food/glucose in the bloodstream) located in the bloodstream outside the target cells. The extra-cellular metabolic substrate becomes permeable towards the inside of the cell. It dissolves into the cell membrane, differentially permeable now only in the direction of extra-cellular to intracellular, and delivers nutrition to the cell. This is part of the active transport mechanism that provides nutrition to the cells.[15]

The Far Reaching Importance of APT Molecule was Recognized in 1997 by the Nobel Prize Committee.

The 1997 Nobel Prize for Chemistry

The Nobel Prize for Chemistry in 1997 was shared by Dr John Walker of the Medical Research Council's Laboratory of Molecular Biology (LMB) at and Dr Paul

Boyer of the University of California at Los Angeles and Dr Jens Skou of Aarhus University in Denmark.

The prize was for the determination of the detailed mechanism by which ATP shuttles energy. The enzyme that makes ATP is called ATP synthase, or ATPase, and sits on the mitochondria in animal cells and chloroplasts in plant cells.

Walker first determined the amino acid sequence of this enzyme, and then elaborated its 3 dimensional structure.

Boyer showed that contrary to the previously accepted belief, the energy requiring step in making ATP is not the synthesis from ADP and phosphate, but the initial binding of the ADP and the phosphate to the enzyme.

Skou was the first to show that this enzyme promoted ion transport through membranes, giving an explanation for nerve cell ion transport as well as fundamental properties of all living cells. He later showed that the phosphate group that is ripped from ATP binds to the enzyme directly. This enzyme is capable of transporting sodium ions when phosphorylated like this, but potassium ions when it is not. This is a key to the function of ATP in the Active Transport Mechanism.

The following is from the Nobel Site[16]

Boyer has called ATP synthase a molecular machine. It may be compared to a water-driven hammer minting coins.

The F0 part is the wheel, the flow of protons is the

waterfall and the structural changes in F1 lead to three coins in the ATP currency being minted for each turn of the wheel.

Walker clarified the structural conditions of the enzyme's molecular machinery and thereby verified Boyer's mechanism. The crystallographic structure of the F1 part of ATP synthase from cows, determined chiefly in collaboration with the Dutchman, J.P. Abrahams and the Englishman, A. Leslie, shows partly that the alpha and beta sub-units are related in terms of structure and evolution and partly that they have clearly differing structures and therefore differing abilities to bind ADP and ATP. The gamma sub-unit is placed as an asymmetrical axle in the cylinder formed by the three alpha and the three beta sub-units and has unique contacts with the beta units and forces their active surfaces to assume different three-dimensional structures. These results can be interpreted according to Boyer's mechanism to mean that the enzyme functions through rotation of the gamma sub-units. It has been difficult to demonstrate this rotation experimentally but several groups have now succeeded. Wolfgang Junge in Germany used spectroscopic techniques and the American scientist Richard Cross chemical cross-bonding. Recently a Japanese group under Masasuke Yoshida succeeded in visualising the rotation in the F1 part of ATP synthase. They attached a fibre of the muscle protein actin to the gamma subunit, and the beta units were attached to the substratum. Depending on the ATP concentration in the surrounding liquid it was possible to show under a microscope how the actin fibre rotated at increasing speed with increasing ATP concentration.

Nerve Conduction Velocity
The Possible Effect of Increased Nerve Conduction Velocity on Visual Acuity

Increased Fusion of Flickering Light by the Retina[17]

When a visual image or a flash of light reaches the retina, it excites the visual receptors for up to 1/10 second. Because of this persistence of excitation, rapidly successive flashes of light become fused together and give the appearance of being continuous. The images on the motion picture screen are flashed at the rate of 28 frames per second.

At low intensity, fusion can occur when the flicker rate is as low as 5 or 6 flashes per second while in bright illumination, the critical frequency for fusion can rise up as high as 60 flashes per second.

The sensitive portions of both the rods and cones contain light sensitive chemicals, which decompose on exposure to light. The decomposition products in turn stimulate the cell membranes of the rods and cones, eliciting nerve impulses that are then transmitted into the nervous system and to the brain where they are interpreted as images.

The Relationship of Resolution and Refresh (JSR)

Consider your computer monitor. A relatively high-resolution monitor will have approximately from 600 X 800 or 768 X 1024, to rarely more than 1920 X 1200 pixels. This is a pixel count of 480,000 to about 2.3 million pixels. That is pretty good.

In your macula, which is about 1 square millimeter in size, you have about 120 million rods and 7-8 million cones. Each rod and each cone is a pixel. At 128 million pixels, that is about 40 to nearly 300 times more pixels than a very high-resolution monitor. And, even more amazing, the comparison of the real estate population density. A 19 inch monitor has about 175 inches square, or 1131 cm² or 1.1 million square millimeters surface area. 1.131 million times more surface than the macula. And 1% of the number of pixels. The macula has a pixel surface density of about 100 million times greater than a high resolution monitor.

A better comparison would be to the new CCD Filmless cameras. The latest SONY CCD, has a ½ inch (8.93 mm diagonal), 3.24 million pixel CCD (equivalent of the camera's retina). This is the highest resolution CCD currently available commercially in quantity. It produces very high quality photographs, adequate in quality for the cover of life magazine. Yet, it has only 2.5% of the pixels of the macula and it is about 30 times the size of the macula. This is an extrapolated density ration of about 1:2500 (CCD:Macula). The macula is still the more remarkable technology by a factor of twenty-five hundred to one.

Consider your computer from 10 years ago: It had maybe 10 to 50% of the resolution of your current system. And you can see the difference. That is why you upgraded. Now you have more detail, faster refresh times, and shorter latencies. All of these details are critical for having the smoothest viewing.

Think about your ability to view video clips or AVI or quicktime clips a just a few years ago. Technology which was borderline pathetic is now coming of age. Images can now refresh at a rate that is allowing the flicker and tiny picture sizes of 1992 to yield to full screen, smooth action. Remember, flicker rates less than 24 frames per second could be noticeable as discontinuous in normal light.

Age Related Neurological Slowdown
The ATP Connection

Vision is a reflex. As we age, our reflexes slow. Is it then so unusual that our vision "slows" as well?

I suggest that this degeneration occurs is because our neurological efficiency is compromised by age. I suggest that we do not respond as quickly because there are simply not as many cells in any particular nerve bundle ready to fire at any given moment, not that we necessarily do not have as many cells. Simply that not as many as

224

them are in the state of "Ready to Fire". Why?

For one thing, as we age, ATP concentrations diminish. Mitochondrial concentrations per cell wane. Hence, if the primary molecule, ATP, which is responsible for the rapid re-polarization of each and every nerve fiber, is scarce, those cells will not re-polarize or will re-polarize slowly. ATP has been called the cell's currency. We need to keep these cells rich (in their currency) and living in abundance.

In addition, what about the concentrations of ATP synthase, which is a protein molecule? ATP synthase is critical in the synthesis of ATP. Since microcurrent electrical stimulation is capable of enhancing the cell's ability to synthesize protein, possibly one of the proteins which is enhanced is ATP synthase, hence the concentrations of ATP itself could potentially be increased.

I believe that using the MicroStim® on post surgical tissues and scars will increase the transmission of information through the area of pathology. I have seen dozens of patients treated who have reported a nearly immediate decrease in numbness (increase in sensation) in areas that had lost sensation subsequent to surgical procedures or trauma.

It appears that this treatment may enhance peripheral neurological competency. A study conducted at the Boston University School of Medicine by Dr. Margaret Naeser and presented to the FDA in

Why not do the same things in the eye? This is the genesis point for another clinical trial, which will have to wait until after the initiation of the ARMD trials.

As we increase the ATP concentrations in the cells, the cell's ability to create the cell membrane potential increases in direct proportion to the concentration of membrane charge. That is why larger nerves tend to conduct faster than smaller ones, which have a smaller concentration of membrane charges.

Note: The cell, when sending an action potential, does not completely depolarize. Only a small amount of ion crosses the membrane. This is why hundreds of thousands of impulses can be transmitted even after a nerve has been removed from the body. [18]

Action Potential and Nerve Conduction Velocity

The refractory period: A second action potential cannot occur in an excitable fiber as long as that fiber is still depolarized from the previous action potential. This is called the absolute refractory period. The absolute refractory period of a large myelinated nerve fiber is 1/2500 second. Therefore, one could calculate that such a fiber could carry a maximum of 2500 impulses per second. This period is followed by a short period of superexcitability. (Guyton)

Consider what the MicroStim® is designed to do, create an electrical charge on tissue. Using this device to enhance the membrane charge on the optic nerve might have the effect of increasing the concentration of charge on the cell membrane. It will, simultaneously, decrease the electrical resistance on the cell membrane, increasing the flow of the current named the current of injury by R.O.Becker MD. [19]

The greater the numbers of charges on the cell membrane, the faster it will conduct signals and hence, the greater the number of visual signals it could transmit per second. The brain interprets visual intensity and resolution by both the number and quality of the specific nerve fibers that are delivering information to the visual center. The faster conduction velocities which can be obtained by the more highly charged fibers will then permit more signals to be processed in a given period of time, giving rise to a higher resolution - better sight.

Remember, these signals are not only occurring up to 2500 times per second, they are also creating a residual effect in the brain that can last up to .1 second. Each signal is the equivalent of a pixel of information and the pixel resolution is increased as the number of signals per second to the brain is increased. The speed that a nerve transmits a signal is called nerve conduction velocity. More signals per second equals an increased nerve conduction velocity. Since the brain images holographically, individual 'pixels' can be transmitted serially and can overlay the previous signal, increasing the signal strength before the previous image fades.

Dr. Margaret Naeser is a research Professor of Neurology at Boston University School of Medicine. She has been the Principal Investigator on two studies using the MicroStim° devices for the treatment of Carpal Tunnel Syndrome. The evidence that the MicroStim° enhances nerve conduction velocity is in Dr. Margaret Naesar's work with the using the MicroStim° 100 together with Low Level Laser at the Boston University School of Medicine.

In October 1999, Dr. Naeser presented a paper[20] for the North American Laser Therapy Association. The presentation was made at the FDA Headquarters, Rockville MD. Table 3 of that presentation presents the Changes in Median Nerve Sensory Latency Times. Of the ten cases that were presented, only 7 could be evaluated because the pretreatment nerve conduction velocities could not be measured. The other 7 patients all showed measurable increases in nerve conduction velocity. The study showed that nerve conduction velocities were increased at a level of significance of .006. There was no significance to the changes in nerve conduction velocities following the sham treatments (p=0.90 (n.s.)).

Possible causes of decreases in nerve conduction velocities

Where are some of the possible retinal/optic nerve bottlenecks and how might the MicroStim® help to resolve them?

1.) Optic nerve bundle cells are present but not firing: Not enough ATP to effect rapid re-polarization of the cells. Stimulation increases ATP, which, in turn, increases the re-polarization rate. In many cases, cells, which were not re-polarizing at all and were so toxic as to be on the verge of death, could be metabolically cleansed and energetically boosted back into play.

2.) Not enough pixels: Rods and Cones and neurological receptors which are out of the game but still alive on the injured list could be energized and brought back into play.

3.) Pixels refresh too slowly: Boosted ATP concentrations will enhance the refresh rate. That is, if the nerve cells are able to re-establish the resting potential more rapidly, they can fire more times per second.

4.) Signal strength is insufficient - Decrease in electrical resistance in the Schwann cell sheaths allows greater signal transmission with small signal strength.

5.) Nerve fibers are damaged - Enhanced protein synthesis may help repair damaged fibers.

6.) Inadequate refresh rate for visual pigments - Maybe we can enhance refresh rates of visual pigments with MicroStim®. Many patients have reported enhanced color perception.

7.) Inadequate concentrations of neurotransmitters - Once again - building blocks of the neurotransmitters rely on ATP for fuel.

8.) Ischemia: MicroCurrent provides smooth muscle relaxation in the walls of the local blood supply, decreases the blood pressure locally, and promotes enhanced oxygenation.

9.) Poor cellular nutrition: MicroStim® enhances glycogen uptake, which is further facilitated by the more abundant blood supply.

10.)   Poor analog signal strength

Becker has demonstrated that Acupuncture points are not simply points of high electrical conductivity but are actually analog signal amplification stations. Using the MicroStim® puts a charge on the tissue and increases the Acupuncture point's amplification abilities. In this way, more signal gets to the brain, even if the Schwann cell sheath resistance is constant.   Add the additional advantage of reducing the resistance in the myelin sheath and you further enhance the amplification characteristics.

Enhancing Resolution

What does it take, hypothetically, to improve visual acuity?

1   Increase the number of functioning Rods and Cones in the Macula.

2   Increase the speed of re-polarization of the fibers of the optic nerve.

3   Increase the rate of regeneration of the Visual Pigments.

4   Enhance the blood supply to the macula.

5   Increase cellular nutrition.

6   Boost signal strength and/or decrease resistance to signal transmission.

7   Increase the concentrations and refresh rates of the visual neurotransmitters.

8   Increase optic nerve conduction velocity.

How these all add up. : The more signal gets to the brain, the higher the signal to noise ratio of visual information. The ways that the signal can be boosted are:

1)   increased nerve conduction velocity = more signals per second = more frames per second = less flicker.

2)   Lower Schwann Cell Membrane resistance = greater amplitude of the analog current signal.

3)   Decreased toxicity of the rods and cones = more individuals signals transmitting information. Etc. That is, every change which increases the amplitude, clarity, and speed of transmission increases the resolution of the perceived signal.

4)   Decrease the electrical resistance in the Schwann Cell Sheaths. This increases signal to noise ratio and delivers more and cleaner signals to the brain.

Are all of these functions enhanced by MicroStim® stimulation?

It's too soon to say, but I believe that most, if not all, of the above hypotheses can eventually be proven.

The analog event: Most of the nerve cells (other than satellite and glial cells) are myelinated. This means that they are surrounded by a material which is lipoid by nature and covers the whole body of the cell. This material is called myelin. Myelin is the main ingredient of the structure surrounding almost every nerve cell that is known as the Schwann Cell Sheath.

When I was in school, I was taught that the Schwann Cell Sheath's only purpose was the isolation (insulation) of one nerve cell from another. Robert O. Becker MD, demonstrated that there is at least one more very important function, an information transmission conduit.[21] There is a measurable analog signal (a small DC current) which flows through each Schwann Cell Sheath. Working with rat bone fractures and surgically severed nerves, Dr. Becker demonstrated that this signal carries information which can direct the healing process and carry RNA coding to different parts of the body to both affect and effect healing.

MS and ALS patients demonstrate the devastating effects of the loss of myelin sheath. This would happen, of course, if the insulation broke down, but the effects are much more complex than that. These sheaths carry the information that guides the healing and many other functions of the body.[22]

It is possible for electrical resistance to build up in the Schwann Cell Sheaths and block the transmission of the analog signal, which is a very tiny dc current. In the presence of excess resistance, the signal cannot make the entire trip from the input to the brain. I need more information about whether or not Drusen is present in the myelin sheath, but if it is, drusen, of course, has a higher resistance than the myelin which is designed to carry the signal and hence would slow down the transmission of information.

The more commonly accepted transmission method in the nervous system is via a wave of depolarization of the nerve cell membrane which is known as an action potential. What depolarizes? There is a **concentration gradient** across the cell membrane which consists primarily of an excess of Na+ ion outside the cell and an excess of K+ ion inside the cell. There is also some interference of the movement of these ions by calcium ion at the cell membrane. Since the depolarization of a nerve either occurs or it does not, this is considered to be a digital signal.

The concentration gradient is created by the active transport of Sodium out of the cell and Potassium into the cell with energy supplied by the ATP breakdown reaction at the cell membrane. When there is more of an ion on one side of a semi-permeable membrane, this is known as a concentration gradient. The active movement of the two ions in opposite directions to create a concentration gradient takes time. It is called re-polarization. The more ATP is present to do the work, the shorter that time is.

The period of re-polarization is called the refractory period and is further divided into the absolute refractory and the relative refractory phases of re-polarization. During the absolute refractory phase, the nerve cell is re-polarizing, but has not reached the state where the nerve can fire (resting potential). It is ABSOLUTELY REFRACTORY to firing no matter how intense the stimulus. If there is not adequate energy in the cell to move past the absolute refractory phase, the nerve will not fire. It will not carry any signal to or from the brain.

The absolute refractory (AR) stage is followed by the relative refractory (RR) stage. During the relative refractory stage, the cell will fire, but a larger than normal stimulus must be applied to create the action potential. If there is not enough ATP in the specific optic nerve for the cell to reach the full resting potential rapidly, it may not fire in the presence of normal light. Hence, if there is a deficiency of internal ATP in the optic nerve, many of the optic nerve bundle fibers will remain in the relative refractory state, (the number of photons equals the intensity of stimulation) so the patient might be able to read in very bright light because the increased intensity of the stimulation overcomes the relative refractory condition and evokes an action potential.

I believe that we can treat the disease at this junction. If MicroStim® increases the concentration of ATP in the optic nerve fibers, this increases the speed at which the cells can reach the state of complete readiness (a resting potential). It also increases overall the number of cells that are capable of reaching this ready state. Hence, if we have more fibers ready to accept a signal at any given time and they are able to get back to this ready state more quickly, we have a more competent retina, capable of sending more signal with less information. Hence, better vision.

As time moves on and the disease (ARMD) progresses, more cells enter, but do not emerge from the relative refractory state. Hence, larger and larger luminosity is required for the patient to maintain status quo of visual acuity. Time moves on, more and more optic nerve fibers remain in the absolutely refractory state. These cells will not fire, no matter how bright the light and relative and then absolute blindness ensues.

The lower the intracellular [ATP] (concentration of ATP), the more slowly the nerve fibers will pass through the refractory stages into the resting potential state and the smaller the number (percentage) of cells which is available to transmit information at any given moment. Conversely, an adequate intracellular [ATP] will provide a resting potential state most rapidly, enhancing vision by transmitting more data more rapidly and hence allowing better perception with less magnification and in lower light. There are estimated to be about 1.5 million nerve cells in the optic nerve. Of these, nearly one million are in the macula, the more of these cells which can be kept in the ready state, the better will be the vision at any given luminosity.

Drusen

Where do you suppose drusen comes from, why is it there, and why is it generally age related?

This hyaline material (Drusen) is apparently made up of at least 11 different proteins[23]

I propose that Drusen is an accumulation of intra-cellular garbage, mostly proteins, including the various breakdown product from the retinal pigments. These waste products precipitate and aggregate from cellular solution when the individual proteins and proteinaceous residue becomes hyper-concentrated in solution in the cell because of the cell's inability to take out the trash. Poor housekeeping because of inadequate resources results in an unmanageable concentration of intra-cellular protein byproducts.

Remember that ATP concentration must be adequate to provide the energy at the cell membrane to create the differential permeability necessary to move the waste products out of the cell. It has been postulated that there is an auto-immune response at work here. I propose that if there is an autoimmune response, it results from and is not the cause of this accumulation of antigenic material. These protein byproducts needed to be properly flushed from cells, which had produced them

236

in the normal course of events.

The math is quite simple. Each cell holds an electrical charge and is electrically polarized. A body cell, like a battery, when it has no charge, is dead. An inadequately charged cell cannot manufacture ATP. A cell deficient in ATP can not rid itself of metabolic waste. A nerve cell deficient in ATP cannot re-establish membrane potential and hence cannot fire or fires only when stimulated with an abnormally high signal. A nerve cell deficient in ATP will have a decreased nerve conduction velocity.

The life of every cell is dynamic. Proteins and inclusion bodies are constantly being broken down, used up, cleaned out and replaced. If there is a breakdown in any part of this process, the cell ages. By this, I mean, the cell becomes less vibrant and less responsive to its environment and less capable of re-establishing its optimal equilibrium state. A cell that is able to continually re-establish optimal performance ages only chronologically. Physical aging is simply the loss of optimum vitality of any cell of the body.

With an aged cell, as the concentration of protein by-products builds up in the cells, these concentrations may eventually reach the point of full saturation. One molecule past full saturation initiates precipitation. Once the drusen is precipitated in to the cells, there is a clumping that occurs and the material is no longer soluble in intracellular bioplasm. The process is similar to the coagulation of eggs in a frying pan. You can not make the fried egg revert to being a fluid egg. Re-establish the cell's charge, bring the cell's ability to re-polarize rapidly and normally back to normal, and you can enhance an ARMD patient's vision. Depending upon at what point you catch the disease, you may be able to bring the function of the macula back to normal.

Fortunately, the presence on the planet of people with large concentrations of drusen and good vision means that the presence of drusen, of and by itself, is not the factor which necessarily diminishes the vision. It may be either an indicator or participant in the vision diminution. but it can not carry out the crime without an accomplice. Eliminate the accomplice and you will stop the crime. Remember, though, that ARMD is a degenerative process. The macula can degenerate to the point that some, many, or all of the cells die. Once dead, there is nothing MicroStim® can do for these cells. That is why many patients will show initial improvement and eventually reach a plateau.

What I am saying is, re-establish the cell's electronic competence and ATP concentrations and you can restore or maintain vision status in patients who have lost some or much of their vision. The prophylactic treatment of anyone predisposed to the disease would likely prevent the disease from ever developing. We would have the equivalent of an electronic vaccine to ARMP. Can you imagine, we could have the first electronic vaccine. There's one for the history books. But that is the premise for another much longer study.

Molecular composition of drusen[24].

Using over 110 antibodies to a variety of extra-cellular matrix-specific molecules, over 1,100 pairs of human donor eyes have been screened for evidence of drusen immunoreactivity. The screening resulted in the identification of at least eleven different molecules that are thought to be primary molecular constituents of drusen. These constituents are proteins that, heretofore, have not been implicated in ARMD or in any other retinal disease. In addition, the sequence of molecular events leading to drusen deposition has been partially characterized. Based on the known identities and functions of these drusen-associated molecules, it now appears that drusen formation is analogous to accumulations of extracellular matrix material in other prevalent plaque-forming, age-related disorders such as elastosis and atherosclerosis. This likelihood is supported by the epidemiological evidence indicating that these diseases are also risk factors for the development of ARMD.

Studies done by Cheng[25], et.al. have demonstrated that introduction of a current in the microcurrent range will have several effects including;

1.) Increase in intracellular protein synthesis (enhancement of regenerative and healing abilities)

2.) Increased glycogen uptake (the building block of ATP)

3.) Actual increases of ATP concentration ([ATP]) up to 500% at the 500 ?A (microAmps) range.

What if we can increase the [ATP] in the optic nerve bundle, increase the percent of fibers in the ready state at any given moment, and increase the intracellular glucose concentration to a normal level in the cells by the simple application of a precise electronic current from the MicroStim®? What might happen? The active transport mechanism would function normally. Metabolic waste would be removed from the cell as it developed. Cells would have no reason to develop drusen. The optic nerve bundle fibers would reach the ready state almost instantly after firing and the vision would be normal or could be maintained at status quo.

What does this mean? What could be the result of these electronic changes?

MicroStim® boosts cellular housecleaning mechanisms.

Proper application of electronic stimulation could have the effect increasing glycogen uptake in the cells of the macule/optic nerve/rpe layer of the retina. This, in turn, would increase APT concentrations which would then strengthen the nerve's conductance capabilities by re-establishing cellular membrane potentials to the -85 mV and increase the cellular membrane charge concentration required at the cell membrane for each cell to be in the ready state to fire normally and have an action potential evoked by a normal intensity of stimulation and operate with maximum nerve conduction velocity. A patient could read in normal light with all the nerve fibers in a state of near instant readiness. With adequate housecleaning mechanisms in place, drusen would not form or, if already formed, it would not continue to precipitate and accumulate because the concentration of protein waste products in the cells would not be adequate to create precipitation.

MicroStim® aids the analog nerve grid.

Yes, there is that one more, very important aspect of the treatment. The MicroStim® is designed to respond to the electrical resistance present in the treated tissue. It increases and decreases its own electronic current and voltage outputs to finesse the highest possible electronic charge on the tissue at the treatment location. The clinical version of the device, The Model 5M (common name MicroStim$^\lozenge$ 400-III) also will measure and provide the therapist with the location of the highest (or lowest) electrical resistance and guide the therapist to add stimulation to the tissue which needs it the most. This will effectively decrease the resistance of the tissue (including that of the myelin material of the Schwann Cell Sheaths) and enhance transmission of via analog information grid. This occurs in two ways simultaneously: 1) By increasing the charge on the cell membrane the resistance to the conductance of the current of injury is decreased, hence effectively boosting the COA's transmission efficiency while simultaneously boosting the nerve conductance.

Appendix: Study Submitted to FDA

Summary:

Theoretical benefits of MicroStim° treatment for ARMD.

1. Increases ATP concentrations in the cells, providing the energy needed to create a normal cellular membrane potential for creation of an action potential. This facilitates the digital nerve net and allows more fibers in the optic bundle to be ready to transmit information at any given moment.

2. Increases ATP concentrations so that the cell has the energy available which is needed to fuel the active transport mechanisms and remove the metabolic waste in exchange for the glucose and nutrients. This will effectively prevent the further accumulation of drusen.

3. Increases intracellular glucose concentration so that the cell has adequate nutrition.

4. Increases intracellular protein synthesis to the cell has enhanced regenerative capabilities.

5. Decreases cellular electrical resistance and facilitates the analog nerve net.

6. Enhances nerve conduction velocity.

7. Relax smooth muscle of the vessels of the retina, normalizing retinal circulatory supply.

Economic Considerations:

ARMD currently affects an estimated 15 million Americans. Because of the baby boomers, the number of Americans affected by this disease will probably double to triple in the next ten to fifteen years. Estimates, in the US alone, are that there will be 30 million affected by the year 2010. $995.00 is the projected list price of the MicroStim° 100i automated treatment devices for ARMD. The cost to society of the loss of independence of our senior members cannot be measured by sheer dollars.

Background Information – Anatomy and Physiology.

RETINAL NEUROTRANSMITTERS[26]

This is not meant to be complete, only representative of the neurotransmitters required for vision.

1. General characteristics.

Today's research on the retina focuses a great deal of attention on neurotransmission between the neurons of the retina. New techniques using autoradiography, immunology and molecular biology are developing specific stains for neurochemicals, their synthesizing enzymes or the nucleic acids manufacturing these chemicals, so that cells containing these compounds can be marked. Cells stained with horseradish peroxidase conjugated antibodies to the neurotransmitters are particular spectacular because they are stained to their finest dendrites and so can be readily classified with their Golgi-

243

stained equivalents. Furthermore, the whole population of neurotransmitter specific neurons are stained so one can understand their topographical organization into mosaics across the entire retina. Some immunocytochemistry for the common rotransmitter candidates has been performed on the human retina (Davanger, 1992; Crooks and Kolb, 1992) but more has been done in the monkey retina and so far the findings are the same in general. The consistency of cell types staining across species boundaries, in mammals at least, suggest that most, with a few exceptions, of the neurotransmitters, neuromodulators and neuropeptides discovered in non-human retinas will be present in human retina too.

2. The neurotransmitter of neurons of the vertical pathways through the retina is glutamate.

Glutamate is the strongest candidate for being the neurotransmitter of the neurons of the vertical pathways through the retina, All photoreceptor types, rods and cones, probably use the excitatory amino acid glutamate to transmit signals to the next order neuron in the chain (see Massey, 1990, for review). There was originally some evidence for the closely related amino acid, aspartate, being present in rods but the latest sophisticated techniques of demonstrating amino acid signatures in retinal neurons cannot confirm aspartate as a retinal neurotransmitter at all (Marc et al., 1995). Uptake, release and action of glutamate and agonists upon second-order neurons in slice preparations or isolated cells in tissue culture have also all confirmed glutamate to be the neurotransmitter acting at the first synapse in the retina (see Lasater, 1992 for review). The action of the photoreceptor neurotransmitter upon the second-order neurons is through two different types of sensory channels though. The one type of postsynaptic receptor type is a metabotropic glutamate channel that involves a second messenger cascade and cyclic GMP for activation of the channel (in the ON-center bipolar cell) whereas the other is an ionotropic channel via AMPA receptors and Na ions (OFF-center bipolar and horizontal cell) Slaughter and Miller, 1981, 1983a,b; Nawy and Jahr, 1990).

Photoreceptors in most vertebrates including human, have a content of D2 dopamine receptors somewhere upon there surface (Witkovsky and Dearry, 1991).

3. Acetylcholine.(ACh)

The classic fast excitatory neurotransmitter of the peripheral nervous system, acetylcholine (ACh), is found in a mirror symmetric pair of amacrine cells in the vertebrate retina. In the rabbit such cells have been named starburst cell (Famiglieti, 1983; Masland and Tauchi, 1986). One of the mirror pair occurs in the amacrine cell layer with dendrites in sublamina a (OFF sublamina of the IPL). The other of the pair has its cell body displaced to the ganglion cell layer and its dendrites stratify in sublamina b (ON sublamina of the IPL).

These ACh containing amacrine cells are common to almost all vertebrate retinas and have been described morphologically in human retina too (Hutchins and Hollyfield, 1987; Kolb et al., 1992). Both muscarinic and nicotinic receptors have been demonstrated in the mammalian retina, particularly associated with transient phasic ganglion cells   (Y cells) (Keyser et al., 1989; Hughes, 1991) and effects of ACh and antagonists on ganglion cell responses are documented but not well understood.

4. Adenosine may be a retinal neurotransmitter.

The purine nucleotide, adenosine, may be a neurotransmitter or neuromodulator in the mammalian retina.

Autoradiography and immunocytochemistry for adenosine has revealed cell bodies in the amacrine and ganglion cell layers (Blazynski and Perez, 1991). Probably most of these cells are amacrine cells but some in the ganglion cell layer may be true ganglion cells. In human retina additional cells that could be bipolar or horizontal cell label too. K+ and light evoked release of adenosine can be measured in rabbit and chick retinas. And the vertical pathway neurotransmitter glutamate can induce adenosine release from [3H]-adenosine preloaded rabbit retina. Additionally some effects of adenosine on the ERG generated in the retina and on the activity of ganglion cell terminals in the superior colliculus have been recorded and the information points to the strong likelihood that adenosine does play a neurotransmitter role in the vertebrate retina (See review by Blazynski and Perez, 1991). Adenosine colocalizes with GABA, acetylcholine and serotonin in various retinas. Much more research is needed in this area.

Membrane Transport Mechanisms

It is of seminal importance to the cell that it be able to transport molecules in and out of itself. These molecules pass in and out in one or more of a number of ways (theories). There is currently evidence that the holes are created dynamically, when needed, to allow the movement of the molecular product.

In practice, given the structure of known membrane proteins, these holes are only large enough to allow the passage of small molecules through the plasma membrane, almost always simple ions like hydrogen, potassium or sodium. The ions may pass through the hole or orifice by passive diffusion, in which case the protein that allows this transport is called an ion channel. Alternatively, the transmembrane protein may invest energy, usually derived from ATP, to actively force ions from one side of the plasma membrane to the other, in which case it will be an ion pump.

Given the importance of membrane transport, cells utilize a wide range of transport mechanisms. The mechanisms fall into one of three categories: simple diffusion, facilitated diffusion, and active transport.

Diffusion

Simple diffusion means that the molecules can pass directly through the membrane. Diffusion is always down a concentration gradient. This limits the maximum possible concentration of the molecule inside the cell (or outside the cell if it is a waste product). The effectiveness of diffusion is also limited by the diffusion rate of the molecule. Therefore, though diffusion is an effective enough transport mechanism for some substances (such as $H2O$), the cell must utilize other mechanisms for many of its transport needs.

Facilitated Diffusion

Facilitated diffusion utilizes membrane protein channels to allow charged molecules (which otherwise could not diffuse across the cell membrane) to freely diffuse in and out of the cell. These channels comes into greatest use with small ions like $K+$, $Na+$, and $Cl-$. The speed of facilitated transport is limited by the number of protein channels available, whereas the speed of diffusion is dependent only on the concentration gradient.

MITOCHONDRIA AND AGING

By John Watring
12-4-96

Introduction

Mitochondria are known as the powerhouse of most eukaryotic cells. The process by which they produce this energy, in the form of adenosine triphosphate (ATP), involves the utilization of oxygen at the end of an electron transport chain. The reason oxygen works so well in this capacity is the very reason that it causes damage to other molecules within the cell; it is an excellent electron acceptor. The flow of electrons down the electron transport chain of the inner mitochondrial membrane produces a proton (H+) gradient in the inner membrane space. The oxygen at the end of this electron transport chain accepts the electrons along with hydrogen ions to form water. The presence of oxygen has other effects due its high redox potential (Alberts et al, '94, p.679-80).

The oxygen molecule is highly reactive with itself and other molecules. Some of the dangerously reactive compounds of oxygen include hydrogen peroxide, super oxide, and hydroxyl radicals, to name just a few of the most popular free radicals. Approximately 85% of the oxygen in cells is utilized by the mitochondria (Shigenaga, '94, p.10771). This large amount of oxygen and the corresponding free radicals in the mitochondria takes its toll on this tiny organelle in several ways.

249

"Gerontologists now agree that aging ... is modulated by the interactions of various intrinsic and extrinsic forces" (Yu & Yang, '96, p.1). In this paper I will be reviewing research that tries to correlate aging with the oxidative damage of the mitochondrial ATP synthase, the mitochondrial deoxyribonucleic acids (DNA), and themitochondrial lipid membranes.

The ATP Synthesizing Enzymes of the Mitochondria

ATP synthesizing enzymes have been shown to suffer oxidative damage that effects the efficiency of ATP production (Shigenaga, '94, p.10775). Research has shown "age related changes of the mitochondrial energy metabolism in rat liver and heart, indicating a decrease of the ATP synthase activity, and accompanied by a decrease of the amount of beta subunit" of the F0F1 ATPase (Kroll, '96, p.57). The in vitro transfection of cells with SV40 T plasmids (which have to do with DNA excision repair and binding of proteins of the beta subunit) causes escape of some of the cells from cellular senescence; thereby propagating a continuous cell line. The process of cellular immortalization in vitro depends on the ATPase located near the C-terminal end of the T protein (Kroll, 1996, p.58).

Guerrieri et. al. claim to have shown functional and structural differences of the mitochondrial F0F1 ATP synthase complex in the hearts of aged rats (24 months old) when compared to young rats (3 months old). They relate this to the alteration of cellular energy metabolism observed in aged animals. The accumulation of free radicals and the decrease of antioxidant systems could cause alteration of the oxidative phosphorylation mechanism" ('96, p.62,70). This does not conflict with the mitochondrial DNA mutation theory because the beta subunit of ATP synthase is encoded by nuclear DNA (Kroll, '96, p.57).

Mutation and Damage to Mitochondrial DNA

The mitochondrial DNA (mtDNA), which resembles the circular bacterial DNA, only codes for about thirteen of the proteins that are found in the electron transport chain. The majority of the proteins, approximately sixty, are encoded from nuclear DNA. Both mtDNA and nuclear DNA are susceptible to mutations by oxygen free radicals. This can causes death or dysfunction of the mitochondria and eventual cell death by interfering with oxidative phosphorylation. Frequencies of mutations differ between mtDNA and nuclear DNA.

The occurrence of mtDNA mutations are much higher than nuclear DNA mutations. The levels of oxidative damage to mtDNA range from ten to seventeen times that in nuclear DNA, depending on the part of the body sampled. It has been proposed that this is due to the mitochondrial association with oxygen (Shigenaga, '94, p.10771-2).

Not only do mitochondria have a greater rate of mutation but they also lack DNA repair mechanisms. This means that through mitotic divisions, mitochondrial DNA mutations are likely to accumulate with age (Stephenson, '96, p.1532).

Mitochondrial Lipid membranes and Antioxidants

Lipid membranes are also susceptible to oxidative damage over time. The fluidity of cellular and mitochondrial membranes decreases with age due in part to the changes in membrane compositions and lipid peroxidation.

A diphosphatidyl glycerol derivative in the mitochondria, called cardiolipin, performs many important roles in membrane structure and function. Among them, cardiolipin contributes to the control of permeability of the inner mitochondrial membrane to small molecules and helps maintains the electrochemical proton gradient. The sensitivity to oxidation increases with age and the amount of this valuable membrane compound supposedly decreases with age. This is paralleled by a decrease of the inner membrane surface area, and increased fragility of the mitochondria (Shigenaga, '94, p.10774-5).

Glutathione (GSH), an intracellular antioxidant agent, has been shown to protect the oxidative phosphorylation mechanisms from the ravaging effects of free radicals. This is done by the binding of the GSH molecule to the ATP synthase complex which somehow protects them from unwanted oxidation.

Antioxidants which can be found in foods include ascorbate, tocopherol, and carotenoids. Evidence indicates that protection from aging ailments such as cancer, cardiovascular disease, and brain dysfunction can be avoided or at least minimized by dietary intake of fruits and vegetables that are high in antioxidants (Shigenaga, '94, p.10771). Melatonin, a new face on the antioxidant scene, is a primary pineal hormone that acts as an hydroxyl (OH-) scavenger (Yu and Yang, '96, p.7,9).

Conclusion

Since the mitochondria are the main energy producers of organisms, if they are not functioning properly diseases usually result. The coordinated interactions between antioxidants, ATP synthase, DNA, and the free radicals are in a delicate balance through the early portion of life and gradually go out of whack, causing disease by degradation of the mitochondria. This is what we see as the phenotype of aging.

Of the many different theories of aging, they all have the second law of thermodynamics in common. "The universe constantly changes so as to become more disordered".

Appendix: Study Submitted to FDA

RESOURCES

Chapter Three

Integrated Visual Healing Seminars:

    For information: (510) 357-0477

    IVHGrace@aol.com

    www.visualhealing.com

Book:

    Amazing Grace, Autobiography of a Survivor, Georgetown, MA: Northstar Publications, 1993. It is available at Amazon.com and Barnes and Noble Bookstores. The book can also be ordered through Grace Halloran at Integrated Visual Healing Seminars.

Reversing Macular Degeneration:

    Two-day seminars with Edward Kondrot, MD and Grace Halloran Ph.D. For Location and Dates: 1-800-430-9328

Chapter Five

Contact Data:

    Edward C. Kondrot, M.D. (H)

    200 Merion Drive, Pittsburgh, PA 15228

    (800) 430-9328; Fax (412) 341-0830

    Email: ekondrot@pipeline.com

    http://www.homeopathiceye.com

    Damon P. Miller II, M.D., N.D.

    881 Fremont Avenue, Suite A5, Los Altos,

    California 94024   (650) 917-8530; Fax 650-948-5360

    Email: millermd@flash.net

    http://www.acupunctureworks.com

RESOURCES

Joel Rossen DVM, Ph.D.
MicroStim® Technology Incorporated
7881 NW 90th Avenue, Tamarac, FL 33321
(954) 720-4383   (800) 326-9119
Email: JRossen@MicroStim.com
Website: www.MicroStim.com

Grace Halloran Ph.D.
Integrated Visual Healing; 655 Lewelling Blvd.,
PMB Suite 214, San Leandro, CA 94579
(510) 357-0477
website: www.visualhealing.com
Email: IVHGrace@aol.com

Percival Chee M.D.
Kukui Plaza Mall, Suite C 116,
50 South Beretania Street, Honolulu, HI 96813
(808) 521-6578

Macular Degeneration Center of Colorado Springs,
Joyce Gamewell, Ph.D. Director
411 Lakewood Circle, Suite A109C
Colorado Springs, CO 80910
(719) 633-9782, Fax (719) 596-5580
www. maculardegencenter.com

George Khouri, M.D.,
1411 N. Flagler Drive, Suite 4100
W. Palm Beach, FL. 33401 / (561) 366-8300
www.palmbeacheye.com / info@palmbeach.com

RESOURCES
James Nagel MD
111 Delafeld Street, Suite 314, Waukesha, WI 53188
(262) 542-0860

References:
Becker, Robert, The Body Magnet, Quill, New,
Quill, New York 1985

Tens: Clinical Applications and Related Theory,
Deirdre M. Walsh, Churchill Livingstone, New
York 1977

Melzack R, Wall P D 1965 Pain mechanisms: a new
theory. Science 150:971-979.

Kjartansson J, Lundberg T 1990 Effects of electrical
nerve stimulation (ENS) in ischemic tissue. Scandina
vian Journal of Plastic and Reconstructive Surgery and
Hand Surgery 24: 129-134

Debreceni L, Gyulai M, Debreceni A, Szabo K 1995
Results of transcutaneous electrical stimulation (TES)
in cure of lower extremity arterial disease. Angiology 46:
613-618.

Kaada B 1982 Vasodilation induced by transcutaneous
nerve stimulation in peripheral ischemia (Raynauds phe
nomenon and diabetic polyneuropathy). European Heart
Journal 3:303-314

Kaada B 1983 Promoted healing of chronic ulceration
by transcutaneous nerve stimulation. (TNS) VASA 12:
262-269

RESOURCES:

Cheng, Ngok, The effects of electrical current on ATP generation, protein synthesis and membrane transport in rat skin", Clinical Orthopedics and Related Research, 171 (Nov.-Dec. 1982) 264-271

Newssome DA, Swartz M et al; Oral Zinc in Macular Degeneration. Arch Ophthalmol 1988: 106; 192-198

Michael, OD, Leland D. and Merrill J. Allen, OD, Ph.D., Nutritional Supplementation, Electrical Stimulation and Age Related Macular Degeneration" Journal of Ortho molecular Medicine, 8 third Quarter (1993) Number 3

Chapter Six
Book:

Healing the Eye the Natural Way: Alternative Medicine and Macular Degeneration, 1-877-341-2703, www.nutritionalresearch.net

Chapter Eight
Resources:

[1] A National Institutes of Health Consensus Develop ment Statement on Acupuncture November 5, 1997" The complete document may be found at the National Insti tutes of Health.
Web Site at http://odp.od.nih.gov/consensus/

[2] The point names are given as the Pinyin transliteration of the Chinese name first, followed by an English trans lation of the point name, followed by the numeric desig nation of the point used commonly in acupuncture text books in this country. A description of how to locate the point then follows. (The point locations have been cho

RESOURCES:
sen that maximize the effects of microcurrent
stimulation therapy, and may vary slightly from
the point locations described in modern textbooks
of Oriental Medicine.)
Alberts, B. Bray, D. Lewis, J. Raff, M. Roberts,
K. Watson

References:
Neuringer M, Anderson G.J. Conner WE, "The
essentiality of n-3 fatty acids for the developement

J.D. 1994. Molecular Biology of the Cell. New York,
NY. Garland Publishing, Third edition.
p.653, 679-80,

Guerrieri, F. Vendemiale, G. Turturro, N. Fratello,
A. Furio, A. Muolo, L. November Grattaglino, I
Papa, S. 15 June 1996. "Alteration of Mitochondrial
F0F1ATP Syn thase during Aging." Annals of the
New York Academy of Sciences. 768: p62-71.

Kroll, J. 15 June 1996. "The ATPase Module and
the Process of Cellular Imortilization." Annals of
the New York Academy of Sciences. 768. : p.57-61.

Shigenaga, M.K. Hagen, T.M. Ames, B.N. 8 1994.
"Oxidative damage and the mitochondrial decay
in aging."

Proceedings of the National Academy of Sciences
of the United States of America. 91(23): p.10771-
8.

RESOURCES:

Stephenson, J. 22 May 1996. "A Role for Mitochon dria in Age-Related Disorders?" JAMA. 275(20): p.1531-2.

Yu, B.P. and Yang, R. 15 June 1996. "Critical Evalu ation of the Free Radical Theory of Aging. A Pro posal for the Oxidative Stress Hypothesis." An nals of the New York Academy of Sciences. 768: p.1-11.

Chapter Ten
References:

Connor WE; Neuringer M.; Prog Clin Biol Res; 1988: 282; 275-94.

Salem et al, 1996; P. Mertinez et al. 1992).
Haglunf etal, "Effects of a new fish oil concentrate on triglycerides, cholesterol, fibrinogen and blood pressure" Nutritional Research 1990; 227: 347-53.

Jamal G.A., "The Use of Gamma Linolenic Acid in the Prevention and Treatment of Diabetic Neu ropathy," Diabetiac Med 11 1994; 11: 145-49.

Kennedy AJ et al, Journal of Neurochemistry 1974; 23: 1093.

Orr HT et al, Journal of Neurichemistry 1976; 26:606.

Lopez-Colome AM et al, Journal of Neurchemistry 1980; 34:1047.

RESOURCES:

Lombardi JB, Society for Neuroscience 1981; 7:321.

Rassin DK set al, Pediatrics 1983; 71:179.

Schmid R. et al, Journal of Neurochemistry 1975; 25:5.

Tallin HH et al, Life Sciences 1983; 33: 1853.

American Biologics, Research Institute, Mexico: Tijuana, B.C. Mexico, 1991.

Hayes KC et al, Science 1975; 188:949.

Wright CE et al, Annual review of Biochemistry 1986; 55:427.

Ogino N. et al, Ophthalmic Research 1983; 15:72.

Pang SF et al, Pineal Reserach Reviews 1986; 4:55

Nakamori et al., Chem Pharm Bulletin (Tokyo) 1993; 41:335-338.

Malone JI, Benford SA, Malone J Jr. Diabetes complications 1993; 7:44-48.

Lombardini, Brain Res Rev 1991; 16:151-169.

Petrosian AM, Haroutounian JE Adv Exp Med Biol 1998; 442:407-13.

RESOURCES:

Keys SA, Zimmerman AWF, Exp Eye Res, 1999 Jun; 68 (6):693-702.

Salceda R. Neurochem Int 1999 Oct; 35 (4):301-6.

Chapter Eleven
Resources:

National Center for Homeopathy
801 N. Fairfax, Alexandria, VA 22314
(703) 548-7790
www.homeopathic.org

Homeopathic Educational Services
2124 Kittredge Street, Berkeley, CA 94704
(510) 649-0294

Minimum Price Homeopathic Books
P.O. Box 2187, Blaine, WA 98231
(604) 597-4757   www.minimum.com

Hahnemann College of Homeopathy,
Point Richmond, CA   (510)232-2079
www.hahnemanncollege.com

Desert Institute of Classical Homeopathy
5501 N. 19th Avenue, Suite 425, Phoenix, AZ 85015
(602) 347-7950 www.chiaz.com/dich/index.html

A list of doctors who perform chelation therapy can be obtained by calling ACAM at (949) 583-7666 or visit their web page at www.acam.org.

RESOURCES:
APPENDIX
Referrences:

Personal communication with Drs. Cousins and Margolis at Baskin Palmer Eye Institute in Miami, 1998.

[2] Center for the Study of Macular Degeneration (CSMD), University of California, Santa Barbara.

[3] Cheng, Ngok, Et Al., November-December 1982. "The Effects of Electric Currents on ATP Genera tion, Protein Synthesis, and Membrane Transport in Rat Skin." , "Clinical Orthopedics and Related Research, 171, November- December 1982, pp.264-271

[4] Cheng, Ngok, Et Al., November-December 1982. "The Effects of Electric Currents on ATP Genera tion, Protein Synthesis, and Membrane Transport in Rat Skin." , "Clinical Orthopedics and Related Research, 171, November- December 1982, pp.264-271

[5] R. O. Becker, "The significance of bioelectric po tentials," Bioelectrochem. Bioenerg., 1, 187(1974).

[6] Kroll, J. 15 June 1996. "The ATPase Module and the Process of Cellular Imortilization." Annals of the New York Academy of Sciences. 768. : p.57-61.

[7] Guerrieri, F. Vendemiale, G. Turturro, N. Fratello, A. Furio, A. Muolo, L. November Grattaglino, I Papa, S. 15 June 1996. "Alteration of Mitochondrial

RESOURCES:

F0F1ATP Syn thase during Aging." Annals of the New York Academy of Sciences. 768: p62-71.

[8] Shigenaga, M.K. Hagen, T.M. Ames, B.N. 8 1994. "Oxidative damage and the mitochondrial decay in aging." Proceedings of the National Academy of Sciences of the United States of America. 91(23): p.10771-8.

[9] Stephenson, J. 22 May 1996. "A Role for Mito chondria in Age-Related Disorders?" JAMA. 275(20): p.1531-2.

[10] Yu, B.P. and Yang, R. 15 June 1996. "Critical Evaluation of the Free Radical Theory of Aging. A Proposal for the Oxidative Stress Hypothesis." Annals of the New York Academy of Sciences. 768: p.1-11.

[11] Cheng, Ngok, Et Al., November-December 1982. "The Effects of Electric Currents on ATP Genera tion, Protein Synthesis, and Membrane Trans port in Rat Skin." , "Clinical Orthopedics and Related Research, 171, November- December 1982, pp.264-271

[12] Molecular Biology of the Cell by Bruce Alberts, et al. - 3rd ed., Garland Publishing, Inc., New York & London, 1995.

[13] An Introduction to Genetic Analysis by Anthony J.F. Griffiths, et al. - 5th ed., W.H. Freeman and Company, New York, 1993

RESOURCES:

[14] http://128.252.223.112/posts/archives/mar98/
890683118.Cb.r.html

[15] http://www.bris.ac.uk/Depts/Chemistry/
MOTM/atp/atp1.htm

[16]http://www.nobel.se/announcement-97/
chemistry97.html

[17] Guyton, Arthur C, <u>Textbook of Medical Physiology.</u>,W.B.Saunders Chapter 50, 1967

[18] Guyton, Arthur C, <u>Textbook of Medical Physiology.</u>,W.B.Saunders, 1967

[19] R. O. Becker, "The significance of bioelectric potentials," Bioelectrochem. Bioenerg., 1, 187(1974).

[20] Treatment of Carpal Tunnel Syndrome with Laser Acupuncture, Low Level Laser Therapy.

[21] R. O. Becker, "The significance of bioelectric potentials," Bioelectrochem. Bioenerg., 1, 187(1974).

[22] R. O. Becker, "The significance of bioelectric potentials," Bioelectrochem. Bioenerg., 1, 187(1974).

[23] Center for the Study of Macular Degeneration (CSMD)

[24] Center for the Study of Macular Degeneration (CSMD)

RESOURCES:

[26] http://insight.med.utah.edu/Webvision/

Index

A

Acceptance 40, 69, 87
Acu-O-Matic 78
Acupressure 56, 67
    See also Point
Acupuncture 51, 123, 127-131, 148-149, 151, 159, 264
Age Related Macular Degeneration xi, xvii, 1, 3, 17, 18, 21, 25,
    28, 33, 44, 61, 111, 203, 208, 263
    See also Macular Degeneration
Akabane 129, 130, 149
Alkaline Battery 99
Amazing Grace, Autobiography of a Survivor 49, 261
Amazon.com 261
Amino Acid 13, 80, 177, 178, 197, 221, 226, 250
Amsler Grid 15
Anger 86, 87
Antibiotics 21, 189
Apparatus 110
Arm
  Jue Yin Meridian 139
  Shao Yang Meridian 133, 141, 153
  Shao Yin Meridian 139
  Yang Ming Meridian 139
Arnica Gel 142
Arteriosclerosis 30
Arthritis 19, 31, 159, 188, 190
ATP 240-248, 253, 258, 259, 263, 268-270
Autosomal Recessive 28

B

Bai lao (Hundred Labors) 141
Bargaining 87
Barnes and Noble Bookstores 261
Battery 26, 96, 98, 99, 110, 111, 121, 243
Becker, Robert 156, 238, 262
Benoit, Joan 155
Berger, Herbert 155

Bright and Clear 129, 135
British Fighter Pilots 41
British Navy 37
Buchman, James 29

C

Cataract 1, 16, 40-42, 88, 175, 185, 199, 203
  Surgery 40-42
Caucasians 18
Cell Regeneration 158
Chee, Percival, Dr. 83
Chelation 5, 6, 93, 185, 196-202, 268
  Therapy 5, 6, 93, 196-201, 198, 268
Cheng, Ngok 80
Cheng Qi 153
Chernobyl Nuclear Power 50
Chi ze (Outside Marsh) 139
Chloroquine 31, 178
Choroid 10-12, 24, 199
College of Syntonic Optometry 82
Color Therapy 56
Cones 11, 12, 13, 24, 213, 228, 229, 235-237, 250
Congenital 27, 61, 68
Connector Wire 96, 97, 100, 101, 103

D

Da Ling 139
Detoxify 32
Diabetes 19, 20, 30, 88, 150, 177, 199, 267
  Polyneuropathy 79, 263
  Retinopathy 2, 177, 185
Dietary Deficiencies 12
Ding Chuan (Calm Breath) 141
Drugs
    12, 13, 31, 39, 42, 89, 128, 150, 156, 161, 175, 178, 188, 190, 192, 196, 197, 201
  Toxicity 2
  Induced Macular Degeneration 31
Druse 24
  Drusen 18, 24, 26, 203, 204, 205, 206, 222, 239-248
Dry Macular Degeneration 17, 23-25, 82, 204

E

Ear points 130, 143
Egyptians 2, 75
Electreat 75, 76, 77
Elkins, Mike 155
ERG 28, 53, 54, 252
Eyestrain 1, 185

F

Farnsworth Hue 15
FDA xiv, 5, 14, 40, 44, 89, 111, 112, 113, 124, 203, 231, 234
Feng Chi 141
Fish Border 139
Fluorescein Angiogram 16
Fovea 13
Foveola 13
Frequencies 51, 106, 109, 118, 122, 123, 124, 144, 210, 257

G

Gamewell, Joyce, Dr. 83, 262
Gan Shu 136
Gary Carter 155
Gate of Hope 136, 145
Genetic Defects 12
Giants 155
Glaucoma 1, 16, 88, 185, 199
Governor Vessel Meridian 133
Great Mound 139
Guang Ming (Bright and Clear) 135

H

Halloran, Grace, Dr. vii, xi, 36, 47-52, 55-58, 81
Harvey, William 38
Hayes, Mike 155
Healing the Eye the Natural Way 1, 21, 43, 89, 93, 264
Heavenly Pillar 140
Hereditary Macular Degeneration 17, 27, 33
Highest Yang 145
Hippocratic Oath 4, 6
HMO 35
Homeopathy xi, 2, 5, 6, 67, 148, 183, 184, 185, 186, 187, 188,
        189, 190, 191, 192, 193, 195, 202, 267, 268
Hypertension 19, 20, 175

I

Ignatz Phillip Semmelweis 38
Inflammatory Degeneration 31
Inflammatory Retinal Disease 2
Ishihara 15
IVH program 47, 56

J

Jarding, John, Dr. 82, 117
Jing Ming (Bright Eyes) 151, 152
Johnson, Ken 29, 68
Juvenile Macular Degeneration 2, 28, 68, 90

K

Kaada 79, 263
Khouri, George, Dr. 83, 158, 261
Kiln Path 133
Kjartansson and Lundeberg 79, 263
Knickerbockers 155
Kondrot, Edward C., Dr. xi, xii, xiv, 7, 29, 64-70, 138, 148, 261

L

Leg
  Jue Yin Meridian 134, 136, 145, 146
  Shao Yang Meridian 135, 141, 145, 146, 152
  Shao Yin Meridian 145
  Tai Yang Meridian 136, 140, 152
  Yang Ming Meridian 145, 153
Lew, Joanne 61-63
Leyden Jar 75
Light Energy 10, 12
Lind, James 37
Little Sea 139
Liver Correspondence 136

M

Macula 1, 9, 10, 13, 15, 16, 17, 18, 25, 26, 27, 31, 32, 36, 88, 172, 179, 180, 199, 204, 229, 236, 241, 244
Macular Degeneration vii, xi, 1, 3, 5, 7, 17, 18, 21-33, 43, 44, 57, 62-66, 70, 82-85, 89-93, 111, 170, 178, 179, 203, 208, 261-264, 268, 270, 271
  See also Dry Macular Degeneration
  See also Wet Macular Degeneration

Malapterurus Electrus 75
Mayo Clinic 69, 71
Melzack and Wall 77, 262
Merrill 263
Metabolic 26, 32, 171, 174, 200, 205, 207, 212, 213, 215, 219, 222, 224, 225, 243, 246, 248
Michael, Leland, Dr. 81
Microcurrent Stimulation vii, xi, xiv, xvii, 1, 2, 4-9, 17, 21, 23, 26-33, 36, 43, 47, 51-53, 57, 61-67, 70-81, 85-89, 90-93, 147, 155-168, 183, 185, 195-197, 202, 207
MicroStim® 4, 5, 14, 43, 44, 51, 56, 81, 82, 83, 96, 100, 105, 111- 119, 121, 122, 125, 130, 131, 132, 151- 154, 213, 231-247, 265
Miller, Damon, MD vii, xi, 83, 138
Mitochondria 80, 208-212, 216, 218, 226, 255-259, 269
Montana, Joe 155

N

Nagel, James, Dr. 83
Nearsighted (Myopic) 18
Neurons 11, 249, 250, 251
New York City Ballet 155
New York Jets 155
Newssome 263
Nobel Prize 39, 225
Nociceptors 77, 78
Nogier, Paul 130
Nutrition 9, 14, 20, 21, 50, 56, 66, 93, 164, 166, 170, 185, 199, 200, 225, 236, 248

O

Olympic Ski Team 51
On Death and Dying 86
Open-heart surgery 38, 39
Opsin 13
Ornish, Dean Dr. 19
Outer Frontier Gate 133
Oxygenation 32, 235

P

Pauling, Linus 39
Phenothiazine 31
Photodynamic laser therapy 36
Photographs 16, 229
Placebo effect 6

Point
1: 145, 152, 153
2: 146
3: 139
5: 133, 139
7: 139
9: 134
10: 139, 140
14: 136, 145
16: 141
18: 136
20: 141
36: 145
37: 135
40: 146
Protein 13, 80, 81, 124, 168, 177, 206, 210, 214-227, 231, 235, 242-248, 253-256, 263, 268, 269

Q

Qi Men (Gate of Hope) 136, 145
Qiu Xu (Wilderness Mound) 146

R

R.E. 61, 65, 66, 67
Retina 1, 2, 4, 9-18, 24-32, 36, 92, 93, 109, 175, 176-180, 205, 207, 219, 224, 228, 229, 241, 246-252, 266
  Layers 10
  Pigment cells 10
  Pigmentosa 2, 27, 49, 176
Reuse, Warren 41
Ridley, Harold, Dr. 41
Rods 11, 12, 213, 228, 229, 235-237, 250
Ross, Elizabeth Kubler 86
Rossen, Joel, Dr. vii, 4, 25, 40, 51-53, 81, 113, 203, 262
RP 27, 28, 48, 49, 53, 54, 81, 218, 219
Ryodoraku 129, 130, 149

S

Sclera 10-12
Scott, Jack, Dr. 51-53
Scribonius Largus 75
Scurvy 37
Sensory Retina 10-12
Shao Hai (Little Sea) 139

Shen Men (Spirit Gate) 139
Si Zhu Kong 153
Snead, Sam vii, 4
Sonoma State University 51
Spinks, Mike 155
Stimulator 78, 92, 96, 111, 117, 120, 125, 129, 156, 166
Stress 14, 19, 24, 32, 56, 65, 150, 175, 177, 198, 265, 269
  Management 14, 56, 198
Sugar 19, 21, 163, 168, 174, 186, 188, 216
Sunlight 18, 180, 215, 217

T

Tai Yang (Highest Yang) 145
Tao Dao (Kiln Path) 133
TENS Unit 76, 79
The Art of Seeing 71
The Body Electric 156
The Probe 96, 103 105, 159
Thiordazine 31
Tian You (Heavenly Window) 141
Tian Zhu (Heavenly Pillar) 140
Time Out Mode 115
Tomato 38
Tong Zi Lao (Orbit Bone) 151
Transcutaneous Electrical Nerve Stimulation 76

U

Ultraviolet Radiation 18

V

Valiant Stream 146
Vascular Disease 30
  Retinal Disease 2
Visual Acuity Testing 14
  Field Testing 17
Vitamin A 12, 13, 170-175
Vitamin C 37, 172,

W

Wai Guan (Outer Frontier Gate) 133
Walk Between 146

Wallace, Larry, Dr. 82
Waveform 106, 111, 118
Wet ARMD 23-25, 36, 88, 177
Wheaten Clinic 68, 72
Wilderness Mound 146
Wing, Thomas, Dr. 78

X
Xia Xi (Valiant Stream) 146
Xing Jian (Walk Between) 146

Y

Yang Bai (Yang White) 145
Yin Bao (Yin Envelope) 134

Symbols

49ers 155

About the Author

Edward Kondrot, MD received his medical degree from the Hahnemann Medical College in Philadelphia in 1977. He completed his training in ophthalmology at St. Francis Hospital in Pittsburgh, Pennsylvania and the Scheie Eye Institute in Philadelphia, Pennsylvania in 1981. He maintains practices in Pittsburgh, Pennsylvania and Phoenix, Arizona.

Dr. Kondrot has practiced homeopathy since 1990 and received a diploma from the Hahnemann College of Homeopathy in Point Richmond, California in 1996. He contributed to the Clinician's Rapid Access Guide to Complementary and Alternative Medicine, Mosby 2000, and has written numerous other articles. Dr. Kondrot conducts weekly talk radio shows and seminars across the country for professional and lay audiences on the use of homeopathy, nutrition, microcurrent stimulation, and chelation therapy for diseases of the eye.

He is recognized as a pioneer in the use of homeopathy for eye conditions and is on the faculty of the Desert Institute of Homeopathy in Phoenix, Arizona as well as at the San Diego Center for Homeopathic Education and Healing.

Dr. Kondrot can be reached at
1-800-430-9328
ekondrot@pipeline.com

www.homeopathiceye.com

Notes: